PROSTATE CANCER DIET COOKBOOK FOR OLDER MEN

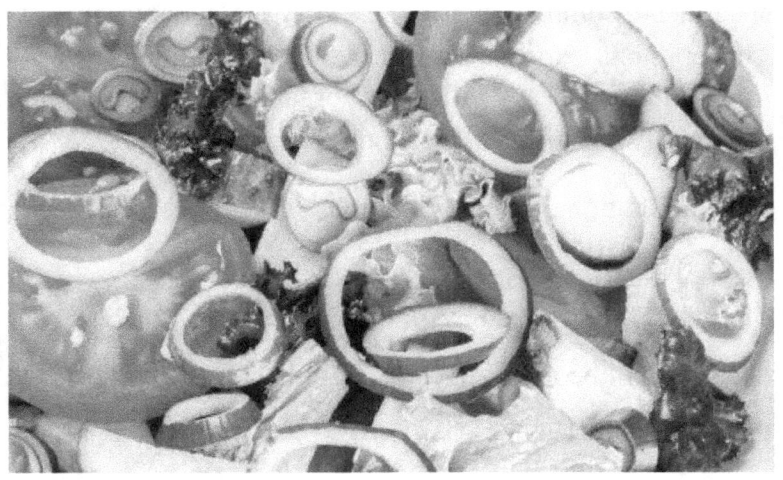

30 Nutrient-Rich Recipes for Prostate Health Management and Support with 31 Days Meal Plan.

Mayer Clinton Jose

Thank you for your book purchase. I assure you that your decision will be advantageous. Together, let's join forces in the fight against cancer!

Gain entry to my additional publications.

TABLE OF CONTENT

INTRODUCTION

As an experienced nutritionist, I had spent most of my career emphasizing the importance of a balanced diet for optimal health. However, my perspective on the profound impact of nutrition took a profound turn when I received a diagnosis that struck close to home—prostate cancer.

The revelation of my health condition served as a powerful catalyst, propelling me into a renewed quest for knowledge and strategies to confront and manage the challenges of prostate cancer. As a nutritionist, I witnessed the transformative effects of dietary choices on various health conditions. Still, the personal connection to this ailment intensified my commitment to understanding and navigating its complexities.

Determined to optimize my chances of recovery and armed with a unique blend of professional expertise and personal investment, I turned my attention towards a comprehensive exploration of nutrition's role in prostate cancer management.

I delved into the scientific literature, consulted with fellow experts, and engaged in discussions with medical professionals to gather insights into the nuanced relationship between dietary choices and prostate health.

My research unveiled a multifaceted approach that went beyond conventional medical interventions. I recognized the potential of certain nutrients and dietary patterns in mitigating the impact of prostate cancer and supporting overall well-being. Antioxidant-rich foods, omega-3 fatty acids, and specific vitamins emerged as key components in a tailored nutritional strategy to complement traditional treatment methods.

Eager to share this newfound knowledge with others facing similar health challenges, I channeled my energy into developing educational resources and support networks. I initiated workshops, webinars, and informational sessions to disseminate evidence-based information about the significance of nutrition in prostate cancer care. Empowering individuals with the tools to make informed dietary choices became a personal mission rooted in both professional expertise and personal experience.

The journey through prostate cancer not only heightened my awareness of the intricate interplay between nutrition and health but also underscored the potential for individuals to take an active role in their well-being. In turning adversity into an opportunity for advocacy and education, I found a renewed sense of purpose that transcended the boundaries of my role as a nutritionist to encompass a broader commitment to the health and resilience of those facing similar health challenges.

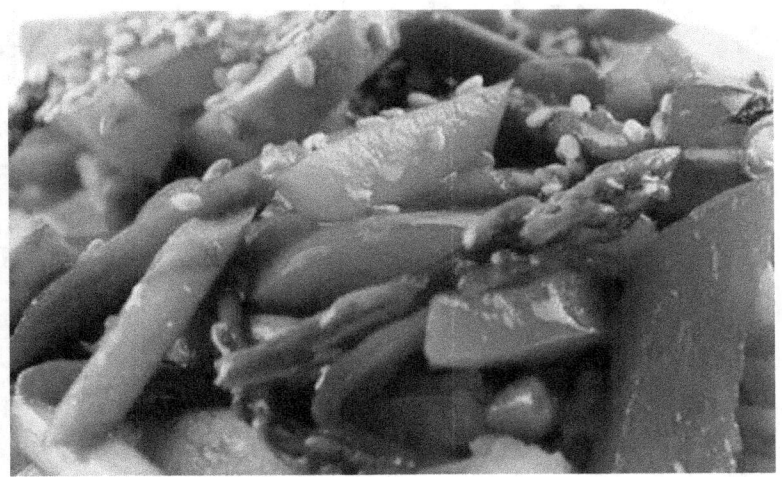

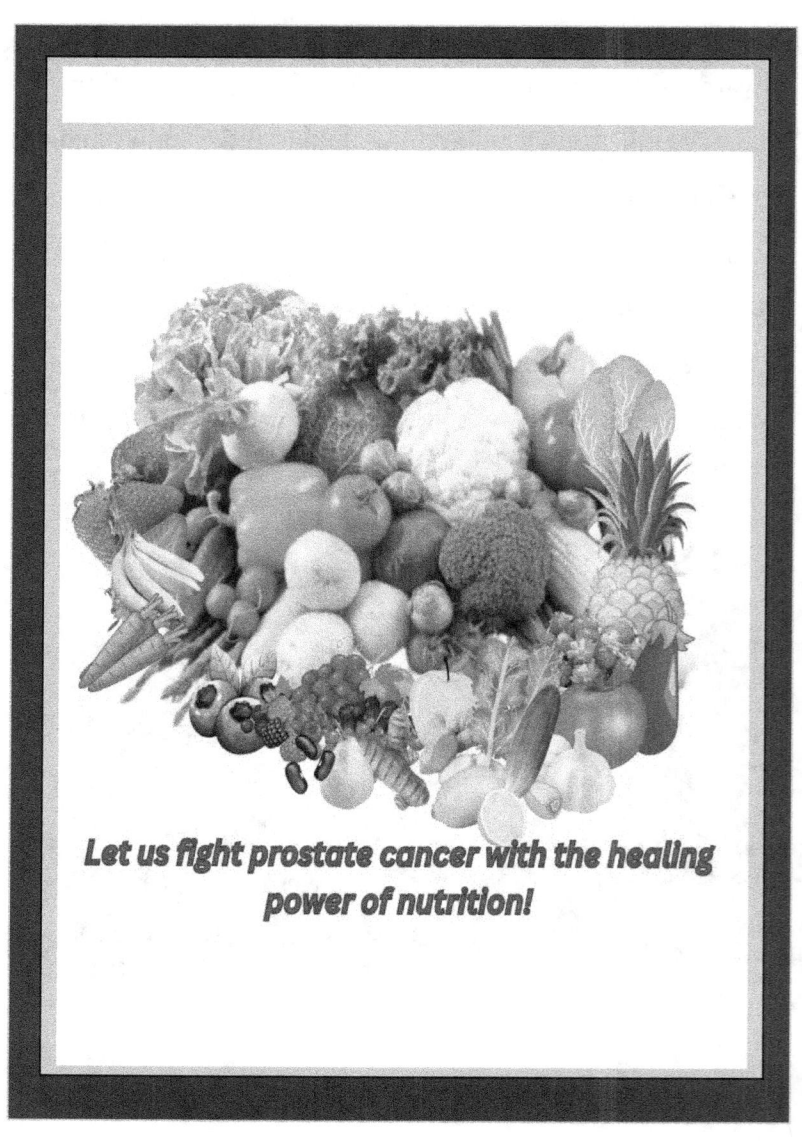

Let us fight prostate cancer with the healing power of nutrition!

CHAPTER 1

Grilled Protein Options

Grilled protein options are integral to a prostate-friendly diet, especially for older men. Salmon, chicken, turkey, tofu, and shrimp prepared through grilling methods offer a lean and flavorful source of essential nutrients. Salmon, rich in omega-3 fatty acids, exhibits anti-inflammatory properties. Chicken and turkey, when marinated with herbs, provide lean protein crucial for muscle maintenance. Grilled tofu is a plant-based alternative, while shrimp offers a low-fat seafood option. These recipes contribute to prostate health and enhance overall well-being through their balanced nutritional profiles.

The grilling process imparts a desirable texture to these protein sources, creating a palatable contrast that adds to the overall appeal of the dishes. The combination of the charred exterior and succulent interior enhances the sensory experience, making grilled salmon, chicken, turkey, tofu, and shrimp nutritionally beneficial and a gastronomic pleasure.

This dual advantage of flavor and texture further underscores the suitability of grilled protein options in promoting prostate health and overall well-being among older individuals.

Grilled Salmon with Garlic, Lemon and Dill

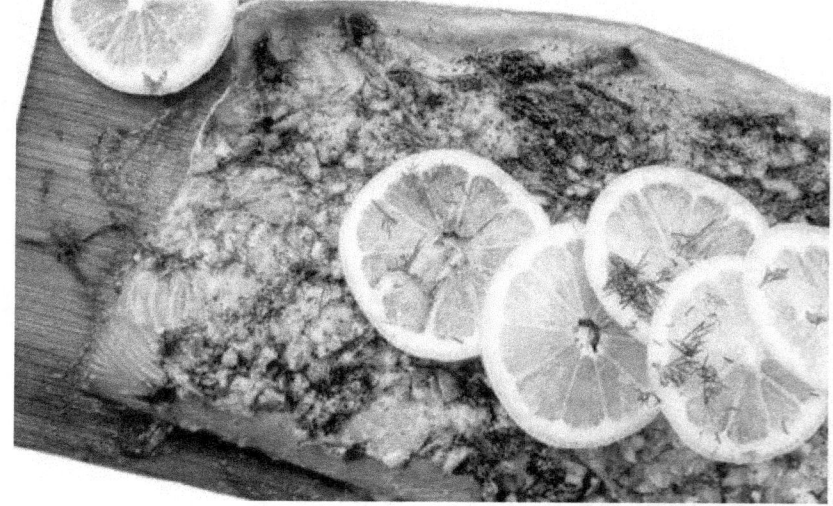

INGREDIENT

- 1 whole filet of salmon (approximately 3 pounds), skin on, scored into serving pieces
- 6 tablespoons of extra-virgin olive oil
- 4 large garlic cloves, minced

- ¼ cup of minced fresh dill
- 2 teaspoons of salt
- 1 teaspoon of ground black pepper
- 1 teaspoon of lemon zest, plus lemon wedges for serving

PREPARATION TIPS

Prep Time: 15 mins	Cook Time: 20 mins	Additional Time: 30 mins	Total Time: 1 hr. 5 mins
Servings: 8	Yield: 8(6-ounce) servings		

PREPARATION STEPS:

1. Submerge an untreated cedar plank (or planks) large enough to accommodate a side of salmon (5 to 7 inches wide and 16 to 20 inches long) in water, ensuring it remains submerged by placing a weight, such as a brick, on top. Allow soaking for a period ranging from 30 minutes to 24 hours.

2. When ready to grill, ignite a charcoal fire in half the grill or set grill burners high for 10 minutes. Simultaneously, combine olive oil, minced garlic, dill, salt, pepper, and lemon zest. Rub this mixture over the salmon, ensuring it coats the entire surface, including the scored areas.

3. Place the soaked cedar plank on the hot grill grate, close the lid, and observe until the wood emits smoke, approximately 5 minutes. Transfer the salmon onto the heated plank, shifting it away from direct charcoal heat or reducing burner intensity to low. Cook covered until the salmon achieves an opaque consistency throughout, reaching an internal temperature of 130 degrees Fahrenheit when measured with a meat thermometer inserted into the thickest section. This typically takes 20 to 25 minutes or longer, depending on the thickness of the salmon and grill temperature.

4. Allow the cooked salmon to rest for 5 minutes before serving. Accompany the dish with lemon wedges for added flavor.

Lemon Garlic Grilled Chicken Breast

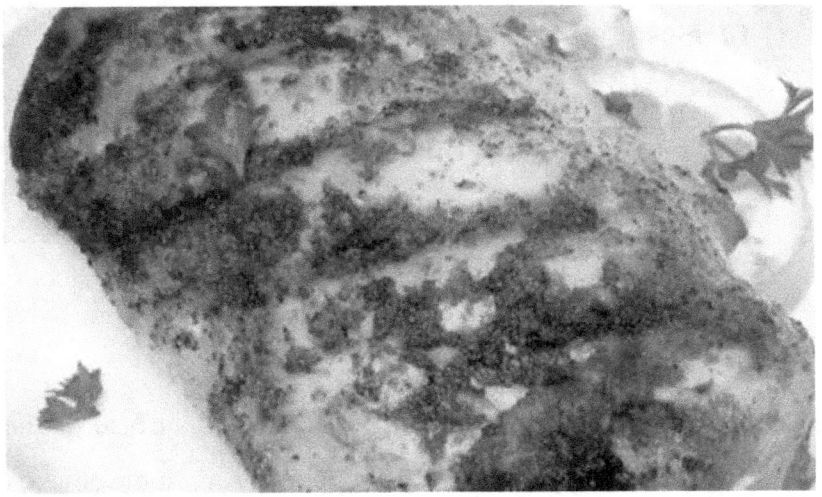

INGREDIENT:

- 4 skinless, boneless chicken breasts
- 2 lemons, cut into wedges
- 1 teaspoon of salt
- 1 teaspoon of garlic powder
- ½ teaspoon of paprika
- ½ teaspoon of ground black pepper
- ¼ cup of unsalted butter, melted, divided

PREPARATION TIPS

Prep Time: 10 mins	Cook Time: 20 mins	Total Time: 30 mins
Servings: 4	Yield: 4 servings	

INSTRUCTIONS:

1. Employ a knife or fork to puncture the surface of the chicken comprehensively. Apply pressure to the chicken pieces on all facets using the cut surfaces of lemons, extracting and reserving a portion of the juice for subsequent grilling.

2. In a mixing bowl, amalgamate salt, garlic, paprika, and pepper. Coat the chicken with half the melted butter, then sprinkle half the seasoning mix.

3. Preheat an outdoor grill to medium heat and lightly oil the grate to prevent sticking.

4. Grill the chicken on the preheated grill for an initial duration of 7 to 10 minutes. Subsequently, flip the chicken, dispense the remaining lemon juice over the chicken, apply the remaining butter, and distribute the remaining portion of the seasoning mix. Continue grilling until the chicken is no longer pink in the centers and its juices run clear, typically requiring an additional 8 to 10 minutes. Confirm the doneness by inserting an instant-read thermometer into the center, ensuring a minimum reading of 165 degrees F (74 degrees C).

5. Conclude the cooking process and serve.

Note:

An alternative to butter is margarine; instead of using 2 whole lemons, 6 tablespoons of lemon juice can be utilized.

When using a George Foreman Grill, halve the specified cooking time for optimal.

Herb-Marinated Turkey Burgers

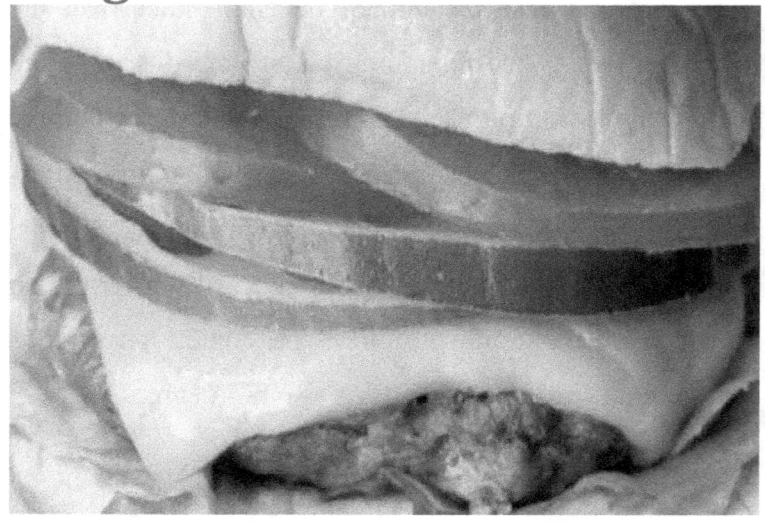

List of Ingredients:

- 1 pound of ground turkey (93% lean, 7% fat)
- 1 tablespoon of chopped fresh parsley
- 1½ teaspoons of chopped fresh thyme
- 1 tablespoon of chopped fresh cilantro
- 1 tablespoon of minced garlic
- 2 tablespoons of grated onion
- 1 tablespoon of olive oil
- 1 teaspoon of liquid smoke

- 3/4 teaspoon of sea salt
- 1/2 teaspoon of cracked black pepper
- 1/2 teaspoon of paprika
- 1/8 teaspoon of cayenne pepper
- 3 tablespoons of butter, chopped into small pieces
- 1/4 cup of water

INSTRUCTION

1. In a large bowl, combine parsley, thyme, cilantro, garlic, onion, olive oil, liquid smoke, salt, black pepper, paprika, and cayenne pepper. Add butter pieces and gently stir in ground turkey until well mixed (be cautious not to over-stir).

2. Shape the mixture into four equal-sized patties. Cover and refrigerate for a minimum of 30 minutes, allowing the garlic and herb flavors to intensify.

3. Create a mixture of water and Worcestershire sauce, setting it aside. Heat a big non-stick skillet over medium heat.

4. Add a small amount of olive oil and the water-Worcestershire mixture to the skillet. Please bring it to a simmer, and carefully place the turkey patties in the skillet. Optionally, make a small indentation in the center of each patty to prevent puffing.

5. Cover the skillet and let the patties simmer for about 10-12 minutes. Uncover and pour off excess fat and juice, retaining 1-2 tablespoons in the skillet. Continue cooking until the burgers are done, flipping them halfway once the undersides are browned. Ensure the internal temperature reaches at least 165°F, adjusting the heat if needed.

6. Drain the cooked burgers on paper towels, and serve them on potato buns with your chosen toppings.

NOTE:

You can make this recipe several times without draining the liquid. It turns out really juicy and tasty, but it doesn't get very brown that way. To get more color, you can pour off the juices. Another option is to cook it entirely in the juices and then sear it, giving you a juicy turkey burger with a nice browned exterior.

Balsamic Glazed Grilled Tofu

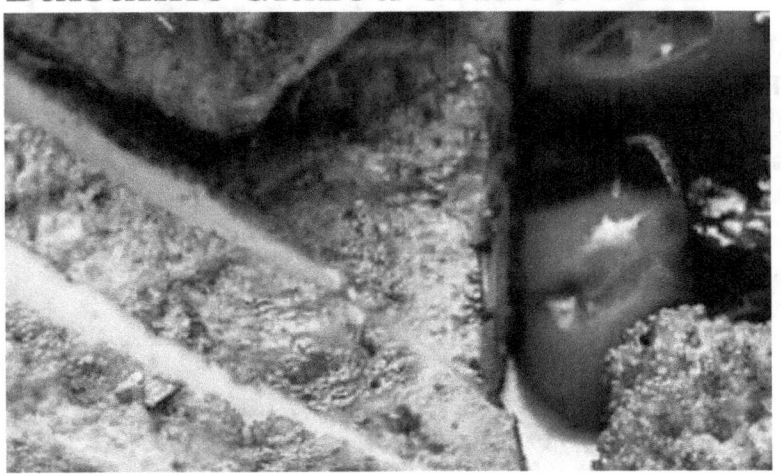

Ingredients:

- 1 block of extra-firm tofu
- 1/4 cup of balsamic vinegar (preferably aged)
- 2 tablespoons of low-sodium soy sauce
- 1 tablespoon of olive oil
- Maple syrup or honey
- 1 teaspoon of Dijon mustard
- 2 cloves of garlic, minced
- Salt and pepper to taste
- Fresh herbs for garnish (optional)

PREPARATION TIPS

Preparation Time: Pressing tofu: 30 minutes Marinating tofu: 30 minutes or longer	Cooking Time: Grilling tofu: 10-14 minutes (5-7 minutes per side)	Total Time: Approximately 1 hour (including pressing, marinating, and grilling)

PREPARATION METHOD:

Press the Tofu:

Place the tofu between paper towels and press with a heavy object for about 30 minutes to remove excess water.

Slice the Tofu:

Cut the pressed tofu into slices or cubes according to preference.

Prepare the Marinade:

Whisk together balsamic vinegar, soy sauce, olive oil, maple syrup or honey, Dijon mustard, minced garlic, salt, and pepper in a bowl.

Marinate the Tofu:

Place tofu in a shallow dish and coat evenly with the marinade. Marinate for at least 30 minutes or longer for enhanced flavor. Refrigerate if marinating for an extended period.

Grill the Tofu:

Preheat the grill to medium-high heat. Grill the tofu for 5-7 minutes per side, creating grill marks. Baste with marinade during grilling.

Glaze the Tofu:

Brush additional marinade on the tofu in the last few minutes to create a balsamic glaze. Allow the glaze to thicken slightly.

Garnish and Serve:

Remove grilled tofu from the heat and garnish with fresh herbs if desired.

Serve Warm:

For a balanced meal, serve warm, accompanied by vegetables, quinoa, or brown rice.

NOTE: The preparation time includes pressing the tofu and marinating it for optimal flavor absorption. Cooking time may vary based on grill heat and tofu thickness. Always consult with a healthcare professional or dietitian for personalized dietary advice for prostate cancer patients.

Citrus-Marinated Grilled Shrimp Skewers

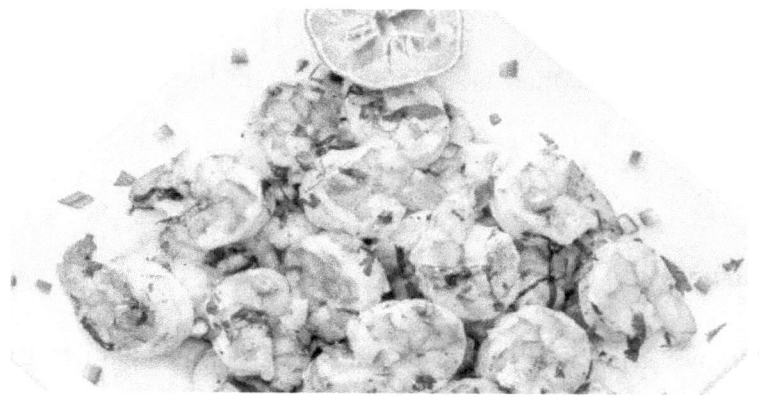

Ingredients:

- 1-pound large shrimp, peeled and deveined
- 2 tablespoons of olive oil
- 2 tablespoons of fresh orange juice
- 1 tablespoon of fresh lemon juice
- 1 tablespoon of fresh lime juice
- 2 cloves of garlic, minced
- 1 teaspoon of Dijon mustard
- 1 teaspoon of honey
- 1 teaspoon of chopped fresh thyme
- Salt and pepper to taste
- Metal or wood skewers; if using wood, soak them in water for half an hour before grilling.

Preparation Method:

Prepare the Marinade:

Whisk together olive oil, orange juice, lemon juice, lime juice, minced garlic, Dijon mustard, honey, chopped fresh thyme, salt, and pepper to create the citrus marinade.

Marinate the Shrimp:

Place the peeled and deveined shrimp in a shallow dish. Pour the citrus marinade over the shrimp, ensuring each piece is well-coated. Marinate the shrimp in the refrigerator for at least thirty minutes.

Skewer the Shrimp:

If using wooden skewers, thread the marinated shrimp onto the skewers.

Preheat the Grill:

Preheat the grill to medium-high heat.

Grill the Shrimp Skewers:

Place the shrimp skewers on the preheated grill and cook for approximately 2-3 minutes per side or until the shrimp are opaque and have grill marks.

Baste with Marinade:

While grilling, baste the shrimp with additional marinade to enhance flavor.

Check Doneness:

Ensure the shrimp are thoroughly cooked but not overdone. Depending on the shrimp's size, the cooking time can change.

Serve Warm:

Remove the shrimp skewers from the grill and serve warm. They can be paired with a side of steamed vegetables or a light salad for a balanced meal.

Preparation Time: Approximately 40 minutes (including marination time)

Cooking Time: 4-6 minutes

Note: This recipe incorporates citrus flavors and lean protein suitable for prostate health. Individuals with prostate cancer should also consult with a healthcare professional for personalized dietary recommendations.

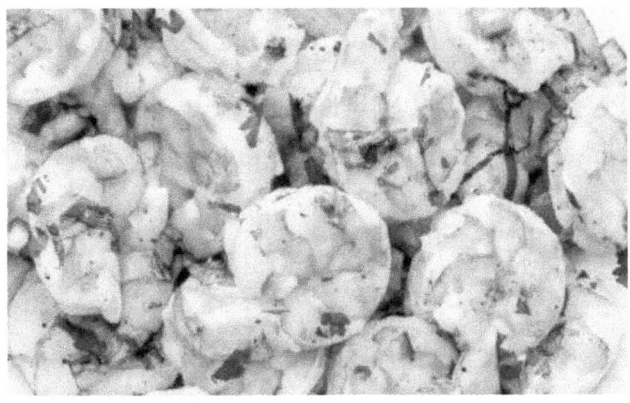

CHAPTER 2

Vegetable-Rich Stir-Fries

Vegetable-rich stir-fries stand as a nutritional cornerstone in the endeavor to prevent prostate cancer. By incorporating cruciferous vegetables like broccoli and cauliflower, these stir-fries provide a rich source of sulforaphane and other bioactive compounds associated with anti-cancer properties. The diverse array of colorful vegetables ensures a robust supply of antioxidants, including carotenoids and flavonoids, which collectively mitigate oxidative stress—a recognized factor in prostate cancer pathogenesis. The stir-frying cooking technique preserves the nutritional content of the vegetables, minimizing nutrient loss. Furthermore, including healthful oils such as olive or canola augments the dish with monounsaturated fats and additional bioactive compounds. Embracing vegetable-rich stir-fries within a balanced diet represents a practical and palatable strategy to fortify the body against prostate cancer by harnessing the synergistic effects of phytochemicals and essential nutrients.

Teriyaki Vegetable Stir-Fry with Tofu

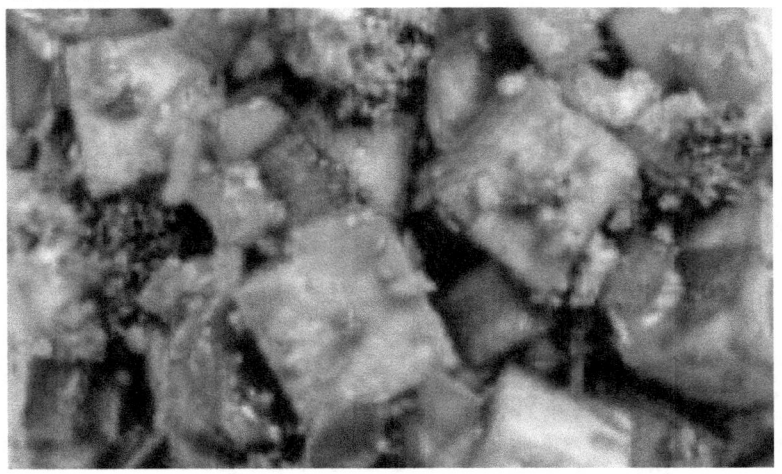

Ingredients:

- 1 tablespoon of canola oil
- 1 small red or green bell of pepper, diced
- ½ medium of red or yellow onion, diced
- 1 cup of frozen chopped broccoli
- 2 garlic cloves, minced
- 1 (12.5-ounce) block tofu, cubed
- ⅓ cup store-bought teriyaki sauce or preferred stir-fry sauce

Instructions:

1. Heat 1 tablespoon of canola oil in a large pan over medium-high heat.
2. Sauté the diced bell pepper, onion, broccoli, minced garlic, and cubed tofu until the bell pepper and onion achieve tenderness and the tofu attains a golden hue.
3. Evenly pour ⅓ cup of the chosen teriyaki sauce or stir fry sauce over the sautéed mixture.
4. Maintain medium-high heat until the sauce is thoroughly absorbed, ensuring the tofu is flipped to achieve an even coating.

Tips for an Easy Stir-Fry:

Broccoli Swap:

If you don't have frozen broccoli, you can use fresh broccoli. Just ensure to steam it first.

Time Saver:

Save time by using pre-made stir-fry veggie packs from the fridge or freezer.

Even Veggie Slices:

Slice your veggies evenly, so they cook uniformly, preventing some from being overcooked and others undercooked.

Softer Veggies:

If you like your veggies softer, cook them for a bit longer and add a splash or two of water as needed.

Customize the Sauce:

Adjust the teriyaki sauce to your taste by adding pineapple juice/apple juice for sweetness and tang, maple syrup for sweetness, tamari/soy sauce for saltiness, rice vinegar for tang, or toasted sesame oil for extra richness and nutty flavor. Experiment with quantities based on your preference.

Ginger Veggie Stir-Fry

PREPARATION TIPS

Prep Time:	Cook Time:	Total Time:	Servings:
25 mins	15 mins	40 mins	6

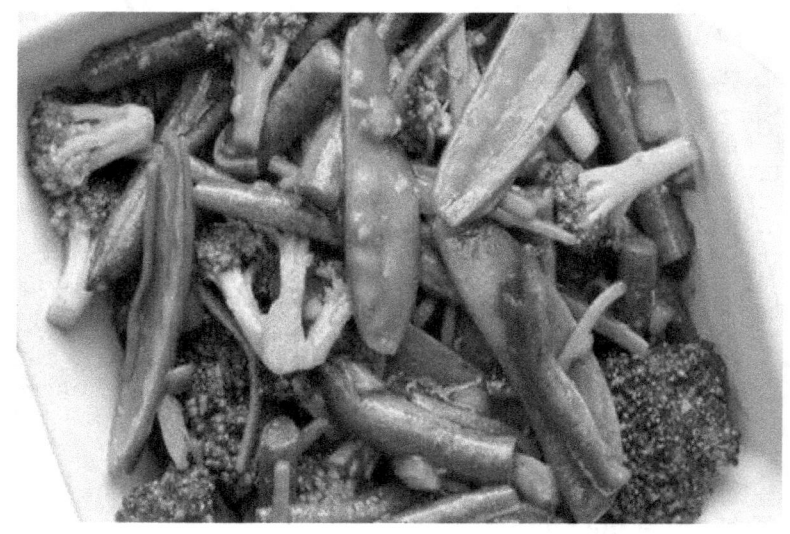

Ingredients:

- 4 tablespoons of vegetable oil (divided)
- 2 teaspoons of chopped fresh ginger root (divided)
- 1 ½ cloves of crushed garlic
- 1 tablespoon of cornstarch
- A single tiny head of broccoli, sliced into florets¾ cup of julienned carrots
- ½ cup of snow peas
- ½ cup of halved green beans
- 2 ½ tablespoons of water
- 2 tablespoons of soy sauce

- ¼ cup of chopped onion
- ½ tablespoon of salt

Preparation steps

1. Begin by gathering all the specified ingredients.
2. In a large bowl, combine 2 tablespoons of vegetable oil, 1 teaspoon of ginger, crushed garlic, and cornstarch. Ensure thorough mixing until the cornstarch is completely dissolved.
3. Add broccoli, julienned carrots, snow peas, and halved green beans to the bowl. Toss the vegetables lightly to ensure an even coating.
4. Heat the remaining 2 tablespoons of vegetable oil in a large skillet or wok over medium heat.
5. Introduce the vegetable mixture into the heated skillet or wok and cook for 2 minutes, stirring constantly to prevent any possibility of burning.
6. Stir in water and soy sauce, and then add chopped onion, salt, and the remaining 1 teaspoon of ginger. Continue cooking and stirring until the vegetables reach a tender yet crisp consistency.
7. Serve the dish hot and enjoy the flavorsome outcome.

Spicy Cashew Cauliflower Stir-Fry

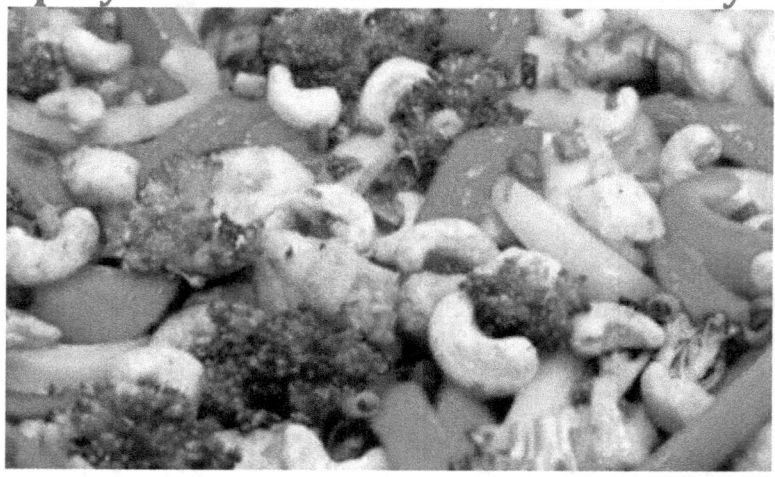

Ingredients:

- Cauliflower florets - 4 cups

- Cashews - 1/2 cup, unsalted

- Broccoli florets - 1 cup

- Bell peppers (red and yellow) - 1 each, thinly sliced

- Carrots - 2, julienned

- Green beans – one cup, trimmed and halved

- Garlic - 3 cloves, minced

- Ginger - 1 tablespoon, grated

- Low-sodium soy sauce - 3 tablespoons

- Sesame oil - 2 tablespoons

- Red pepper flakes - 1/2 teaspoon (adjust to taste)
- Olive oil - 2 tablespoons
- Salt and pepper to taste

Prep Time	Cook Time	Total Time
5minutes min	10minutes mins	15minutes mins

Preparation steps:

1. Blanch Cashews: In a small pot, blanch the cashews by boiling them for 5 minutes. Drain and set aside.

2. Stir-Fry Vegetables: Heat olive oil in a wok or large pan over medium-high heat. Add minced garlic, and grated ginger, and sauté for 1-2 minutes until fragrant. Add cauliflower, broccoli, bell peppers, carrots, and green beans. Stir-fry for 5-7 minutes until vegetables are slightly tender but still crisp.

3. Prepare Sauce: In a small bowl, mix soy sauce, sesame oil, and red pepper flakes. Pour the sauce over the vegetables and toss to coat evenly.

4. Add Cashews: Incorporate the blanched cashews into the stir-fry, ensuring they are evenly distributed.

5. Season: Adjust the seasoning with salt and pepper according to taste. Be mindful of the sodium content, considering the patient's health condition.

6. Finish Cooking: Continue stir-frying for an additional 2-3 minutes until the vegetables are cooked to the desired tenderness.

7. Serve: Remove from heat and serve the Spicy Cashew Cauliflower Stir-fry immediately. Optionally, garnish with fresh cilantro or green onions.

Sesame Ginger Asparagus Stir-Fry

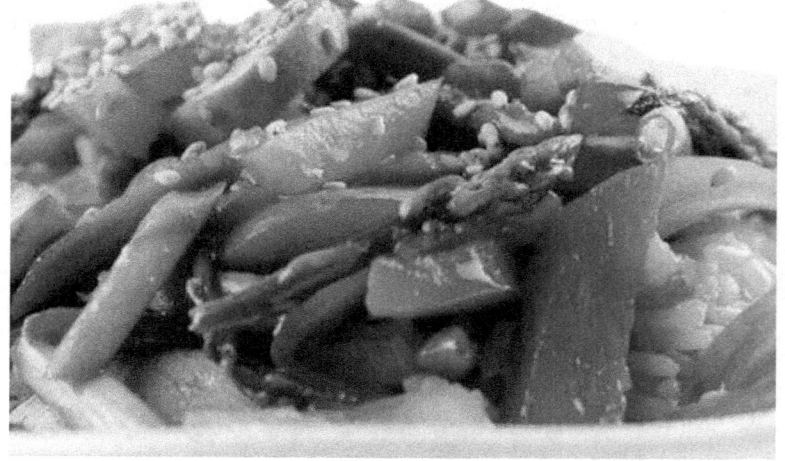

- **Ingredient:**
- 1 lb of fresh asparagus, washed and trimmed
- 2 tablespoons of sesame oil

- 2 tablespoons of low-sodium soy sauce
- 1 tablespoon of fresh ginger, minced
- 2 cloves of garlic, minced
- 1 tablespoon of rice vinegar
- 1 tablespoon of honey
- 1 teaspoon of cornstarch for thickening(optional)
- one tablespoon of sesame seeds for garnish (optional)
- 1 tablespoon of green onions, finely chopped (optional, for garnish)

PREPARATION TIPS

Prep Time: 10 min	Cooking Time 20 min	Total Time: 35 mins	Serving 2

Instructions:

1. Wash and trim the asparagus, removing tough ends. Cut the asparagus into 2-inch pieces.
2. Heat 1 tablespoon of sesame oil over medium-high heat in a wok or large skillet.

3. Add the minced ginger and garlic to the hot oil, stirring constantly for about 30 seconds until fragrant.

4. Add the trimmed asparagus to the wok or skillet. Stir-fry the asparagus for 3-4 minutes until it becomes tender-crisp. Adjust the cooking time based on your preference for asparagus texture.

5. Whisk together the soy sauce, rice vinegar, and honey in a small bowl. Pour the mixture over the stir-fried asparagus and toss to coat evenly.

6. If you prefer a thicker sauce, dissolve 1 teaspoon of cornstarch in 2 teaspoons of water. Add this mixture to the wok or skillet and stir well until the sauce thickens slightly.

7. Drizzle the remaining tablespoon of sesame oil over the stir-fry and toss to combine.

8. If preferred, Garnish with sesame seeds and chopped green onions.

9. Remove the stir-fry from the heat and serve immediately. This dish can be enjoyed independently or paired with brown rice or quinoa for a wholesome meal.

CHAPTER 3

Whole Grain Delights

Whole Grain Delight foods offer valuable nutritional benefits for prostate health. Rich in dietary fiber, these products support bowel regularity, potentially reducing inflammation and irritation in the prostate. Packed with essential nutrients such as vitamin E, selenium, and zinc, Whole Grain Delights contributes to the overall well-being of the prostate and may help lower the risk of prostate-related issues. The antioxidant content in these foods further aids in counteracting oxidative stress, a factor associated with prostate inflammation. Additionally, bioactive compounds in whole grains provide anti-inflammatory properties, potentially mitigating the risk of chronic inflammation linked to prostate conditions. In summary, incorporating Whole Grain Delights foods into one's diet provides a holistic approach to supporting prostate health through a combination of dietary fiber, essential vitamins and minerals, antioxidants, and anti-inflammatory compounds.

Kale, Quinoa, and Avocado Salad with Lemon Dijon Vinaigrette

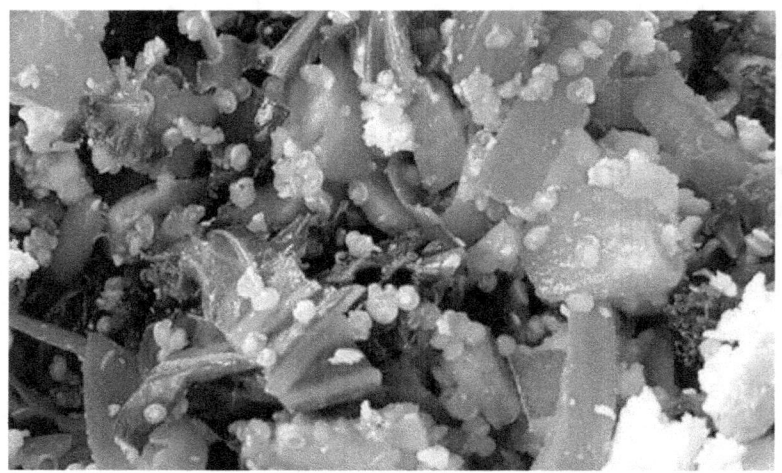

Ingredient

- Two-thirds (2/3) cup of quinoa.

- One and one-third (1 and 1/3) cups of water.

- A single bunch of kale, torn into bite-sized pieces.

- Half (1/2) of an avocado, peeled, pitted, and diced.

- Half (1/2) cup of chopped cucumber.

- One-third (1/3) cup of chopped red bell pepper.

- Two tablespoons of chopped red onion.

- One tablespoon of crumbled feta cheese.

- **Combine the following ingredients to make the dressing:**

- 1/4 cup of olive oil

- 2 tablespoons of lemon juice

- 1 1/2 tablespoons of Dijon mustard

- 3/4 teaspoon of sea salt

- 1/4 teaspoon of ground black pepper

PREPARATION TIPS

Prep Time:	Cook Time:	Total Time:
25 mins	15 mins	40 mins
Servings:	**Yield:**	
4	1 large salad	

Preparation steps

1. Bring quinoa and 1 and 1/3 cups of water to a boil in a saucepan. Subsequently, reduce the heat to medium-low, cover, and simmer until the quinoa attains tenderness and absorbs the water, typically requiring 15 to 20 minutes. Allow the quinoa to cool and set it aside.

2. Position kale in a steamer basket above 1 inch of boiling water in another saucepan.

3. Cover the saucepan with a lid and steam the kale until heated, approximately 45 seconds. Transfer the steamed kale to a sizable plate. Layer the kale with quinoa, avocado, cucumber, bell pepper, red onion, and feta cheese.

4. Prepare the dressing by whisking together olive oil, lemon juice, Dijon mustard, sea salt, and black pepper in a bowl until the oil emulsifies. Subsequently, pour the dressing over the salad, ensuring even distribution.

5. Serve

Whole Wheat Spaghetti with Tomato and Basil Sauce

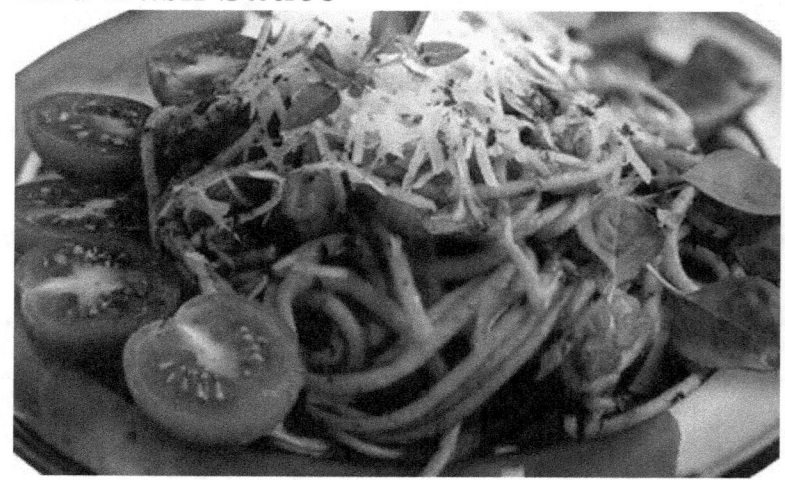

List of Ingredients:

- 100 grams of whole-wheat spaghetti
- 5-6 tomatoes
- 3 cloves of garlic (chopped)
- 2 tablespoons of olive oil
- ½ teaspoon of red chili flakes
- Salt (to taste)
- 1 teaspoon of lemon juice (optional)
- 3 tablespoons of basil
- Grated Parmesan cheese (for garnishing)

Prep Time:	Cooking Time	Serving
10 minutes	20 minutes	2

Procedure:

1. Boil spaghetti in salted water until it reaches an al dente consistency. Save half of the cooking water.
2. In a large skillet, sauté olive oil, garlic, and chili flakes until the garlic turns golden.
3. Optionally, incorporate vegetables like crisp-tender broccoli, bell peppers, chickpeas, etc.

4. Combine the cooked spaghetti and reserved water in the skillet. Cook over moderate heat, stirring occasionally until well mixed.

5. Drizzle with lemon juice and savor the dish.

Zucchini Herb Casserole

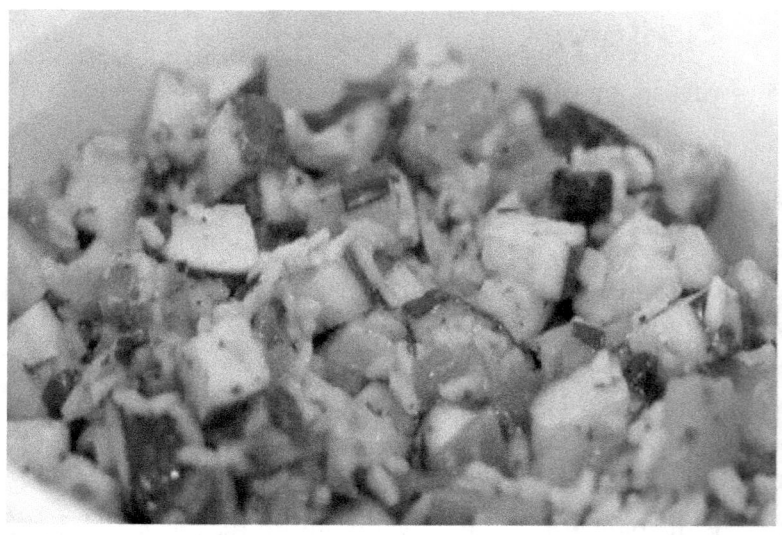

Ingredient

- One-third cup of uncooked long-grain of Brown rice
- Two-thirds cup of water
- Two tablespoons of vegetable oil
- One and a half pounds of zucchini, cubed

- One cup of sliced green onions
- One clove of minced garlic
- One and a quarter teaspoon of garlic salt
- Half a teaspoon of basil
- Half a teaspoon of sweet paprika
- Half a teaspoon of dried oregano
- One and a half cups of seeded, chopped tomatoes
- Two cups of shredded sharp Cheddar cheese divided

PREPARATION TIPS

Prep Time:	Cook Time:	Total Time:
15 mins	40 mins	55 mins
Servings:	Yield:	
6	6 servings	

Instructions:

1. Combine rice and water in a saucepan, bringing it to a boil. Once boiling, reduce the heat to low, cover, and simmer for 20 minutes or until the rice reaches a tender consistency.

2. Preheat the oven to 350 degrees F (175 degrees C) and lightly grease a shallow 1 1/2-quart casserole dish.

3. In a skillet over medium heat, heat oil. Cook zucchini, green onions, and garlic for approximately 5 minutes or until tender. Season the mixture with garlic salt, basil, paprika, and oregano. Incorporate the cooked rice, tomatoes, and 1 cup of cheese, continue cooking, and stir until heated.

4. Transfer the prepared mixture to the greased casserole dish. Sprinkle the remaining cheese on top.

5. Bake the dish uncovered for 20 minutes or until the cheese is melted and bubbly.

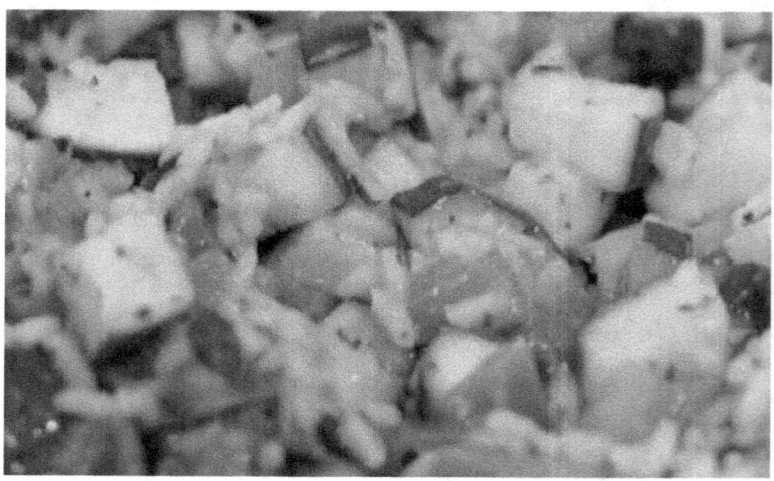

Barley and Vegetable Stuffed Bell Peppers

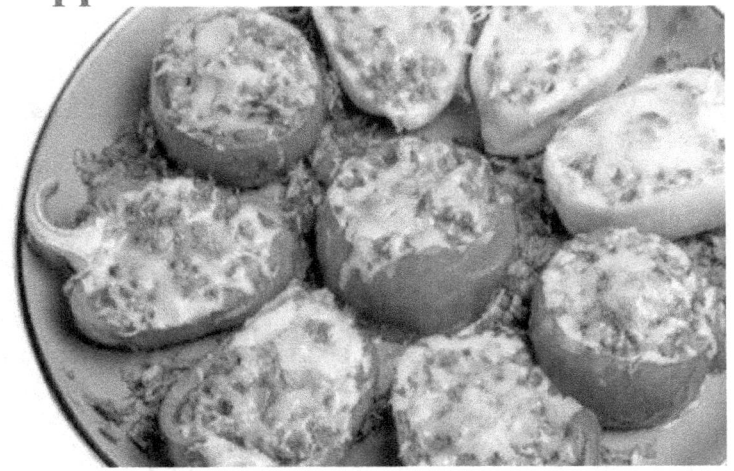

Ingredients:

- 2 cups of cooked barley

- 2 large bell peppers

- 1 tablespoon of olive oil

- 1 small onion, diced

- 2 cloves of garlic

- ½ cup of cherry tomatoes, halved

- ½ cup of vegan feta

- ¼ cup of chopped basil, plus additional for topping

- 1 teaspoon of Italian herbs

- ½ teaspoon of salt
- ¼ teaspoon black pepper

Prep Time	Cook Time	Total Time
15 mins	15min	30min

Instructions:

1. Allow the oven to heat for 375°F or 190°C.

2. Sauté garlic & onion: In a small skillet over medium heat, heat 1 tablespoon of olive oil. Add diced onion and minced garlic cloves, cooking for 3-4 minutes until the onion becomes slightly translucent.

3. Start to boil water: While the onion is cooking, bring water to a boil in a large pot suitable for accommodating the peppers. Add a pinch of salt to the boiling water and prepare a large bowl of ice-cold water.

4. How to blanch peppers: Place the bell peppers into the boiling water and cook for 3 minutes until their skin soften, rotating them if necessary to ensure even blanching.

5. Submerge in an ice bath: Using tongs, remove the peppers and immediately submerge them in the ice water bath for one minute to halt the cooking process. Pat them dry with a paper towel to eliminate excess water.

6. Carve out peppers: Cut the peppers in half and carefully remove the insides using a small paring knife or spoon. If there are any lingering seeds, rinse the peppers under cold water to remove them.

7. Mix stuffing ingredients: Combine the cooked barley, sliced cherry tomatoes, chopped basil, vegan feta crumbles, salt, pepper, and Italian herbs in a bowl.

8. Prepare stuffed peppers: Spoon the barley mixture into each pepper half and press down with a spoon to fill the crevices. Optionally, top the peppers with more vegan cheese.

9. Cook peppers: Place the stuffed peppers in the preheated oven and bake for 15 minutes (uncovered) until the peppers are tender but still slightly firm and the stuffing is warm. Extend the cooking time if the peppers are too firm.

10. Serve with additional fresh basil on top if desired.

Farro and Roasted Brussels Sprouts Bowl

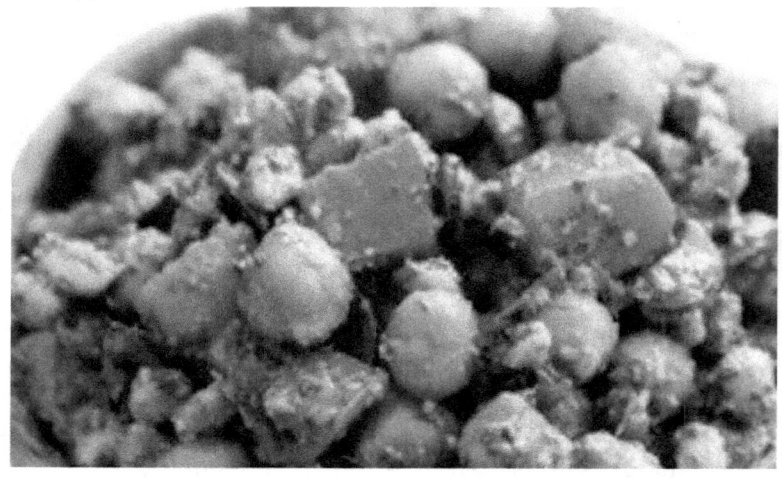

LIST OF INGREDIENTS:

- 1 cup of uncooked farro
- 1/2 cup of chopped pecans
- One pound of trimmed and halved Brussels sprouts
- 1/2 cup of pumpkin seeds
- 1 cup of pomegranate seeds
- 1 tbsp of olive oil
- 2 tbsp of balsamic vinegar (divided)
- 1 tbsp of maple syrup
- 1 tsp of Dijon mustard

- 1 tsp of sea salt
- Black pepper, to taste
- 1 tsp of dried thyme

PREPARATION TIPS

Prep Time:	Cook Time:	Total Time:	Yield:
10 minutes	40 minutes	50 minutes	4 servings

INSTRUCTIONS:

1. Preheat the oven to 425 degrees F.
2. Place the trimmed and halved Brussels sprouts on a lined baking sheet. Coat them with olive oil and 1 tbsp of balsamic vinegar. Sprinkle with salt.
3. Bake for 30 minutes or until the Brussels sprouts are slightly charred.
4. Meanwhile, cook the farro on the stovetop according to package instructions (generally, add 1:2 ratio of farro to water).
5. Place the pecans and pumpkin seeds on the stovetop over medium-high heat in a skillet. Cook until they are slightly browned, watching for potential burning.

6. In a large bowl, combine the cooked farro, pecans, pumpkin seeds, pomegranate seeds, and Brussels sprouts once they are done cooking.

7. Combine the remaining 1 tbsp of balsamic vinegar, maple syrup, and Dijon mustard in a small bowl. Stir to combine.

8. Pour the dressing onto the salad and stir in the sea salt, black pepper, and dried thyme.

9. Serve the salad warm or cold, depending on preference.

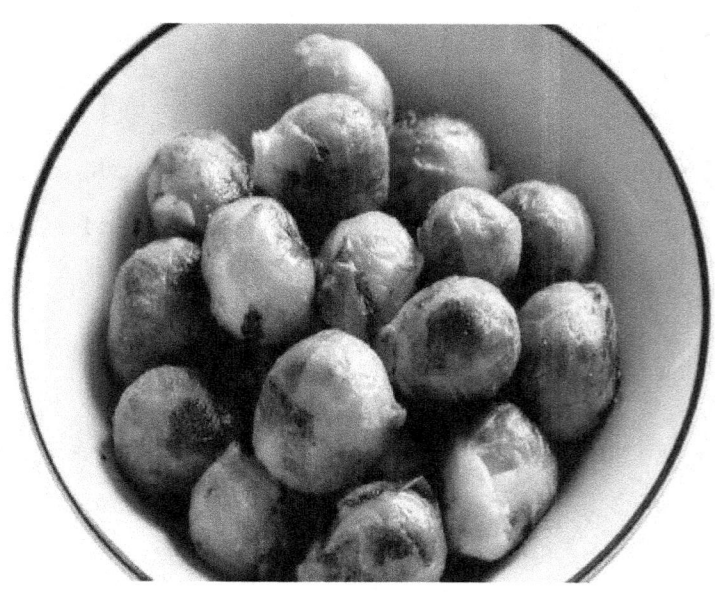

Roasted Brussels

CHAPTER 4

Nutrient-Packed Salads

Nutrient-packed salads are pivotal in supporting prostate health due to their rich array of vitamins, minerals, and bioactive compounds. Ingredients like tomatoes and red peppers, abundant in antioxidants like lycopene, have been associated with a decreased risk of prostate cancer. Additionally, cruciferous vegetables such as broccoli contribute to sulforaphane, known for its anti-cancer properties. At the same time, leafy greens like spinach provide vital nutrients, collectively enhancing the overall nutritional profile of these salads.

Including nuts and seeds in nutrient-packed salads introduces omega-3 fatty acids, recognized for their anti-inflammatory effects. This is particularly relevant to prostate health, as chronic inflammation is linked to an elevated risk of prostate-related conditions. In summary, nutrient-packed salads offer a concise and effective means of incorporating a range of prostate-supportive nutrients, making them a valuable component of a health-conscious diet.

Spinach and Walnut Salad with Pomegranate Vinaigrette

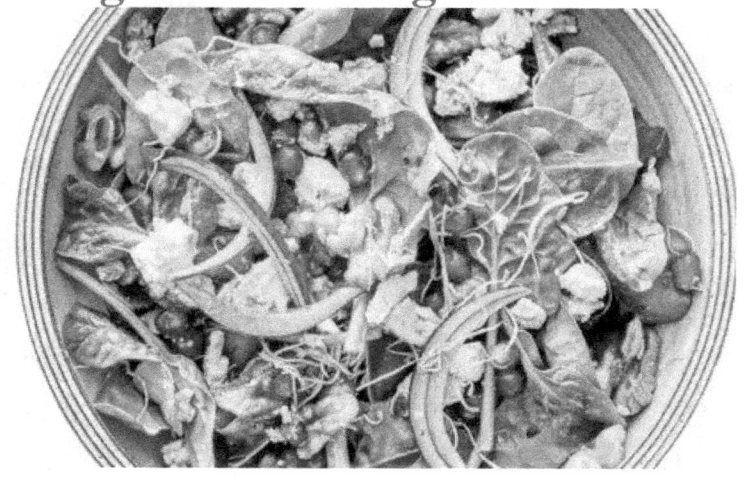

Ingredients:

- 1 bag (10 ounces) of fresh baby spinach leaves, washed and drained
- 1/2 cup of chopped walnut pieces
- 1/2 cup of crumbled feta cheese
- Thinly slice 1/4 of a medium red onion1/4 cup of optional alfalfa sprouts
- 1/2 cup of pomegranate seeds, or adjust to taste
- 4 tablespoons of balsamic vinaigrette dressing

PREPARATION TIPS

Prep Time: 5 mins	Total Time: 15 mins	Servings: 4

Procedure:

1. Assemble all the necessary ingredients.
2. Combine spinach, walnuts, feta, red onion, alfalfa sprouts, and pomegranate seeds in a salad bowl.
3. Pour vinaigrette over the salad.
4. Serve and savor!

Avocado and Tomato Salad with Cilantro-Lime Dressing

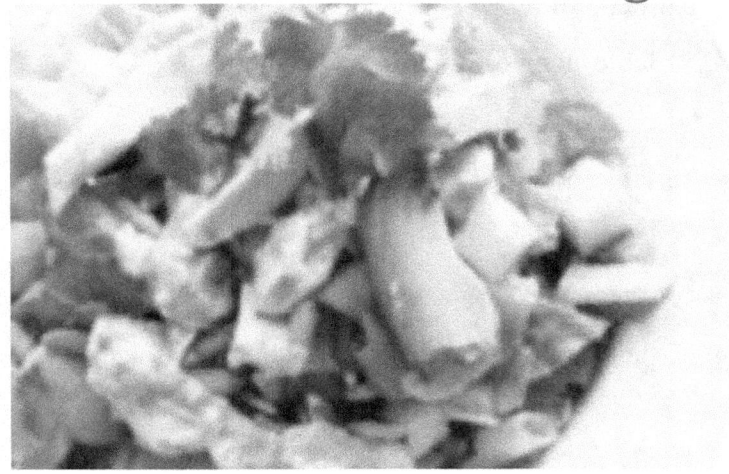

Ingredients:

- 1 head of Romaine lettuce
- 1 large tomato, diced
- 2 ripe of avocados, sliced
- 1 cucumber, peeled and chopped
- 1 bunch of cilantro, finely minced (stems removed)
- 1/4 cup of toasted pepitas
- Cotija or goat cheese for topping (Optional)

Dressing Ingredients:

- 1 avocado
- 2 cloves of garlic, peeled
- 1/2 cup of loosely packed cilantro
- 1/4 cup of light sour cream
- 1 tablespoon of lime juice
- 1 tablespoon of lemon juice
- 3 tablespoons of olive oil
- 1/2 teaspoon of Kosher salt
- 1/4 teaspoon of black pepper
- 2 tablespoons of water, plus additional as needed

PREPARATION TIPS

Prep Time: 20 mins	Cook Time: 10 mins	Total Time: 30 mins
Servings: 4	Yield: 4 servings	

Instruction:

1. Gather all the ingredient
2. Combine all the salad ingredients in a big bowl, leaving out the pepitas and cheese.
3. Use a food processor to blend the dressing ingredients until they're smooth.
4. If needed, add water gradually (1 tablespoon at a time) until you get the thickness you want.
5. Share the mixed salad in bowls and sprinkle pepitas, dressing, and cheese on top.
6. Serve and enjoy!

Kale Caesar Salad with Grilled Chicken

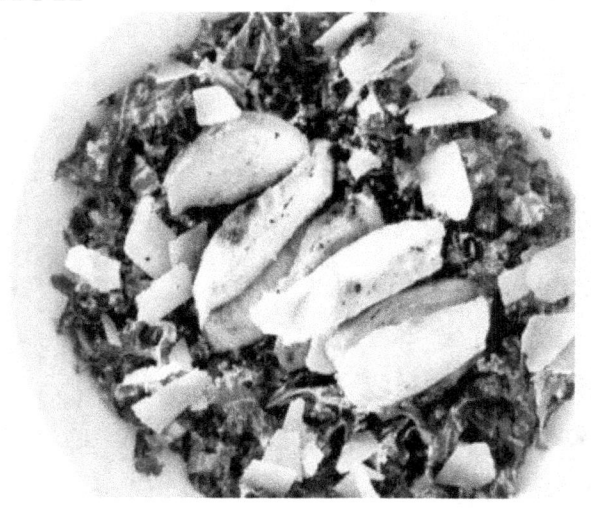

Ingredients:

- 2 curly kale leaves
- 4 oz. chicken breast
- Shaved parmesan
- Salt
- Pepper
- **For the dressing:**
- 1 tbsp mayonnaise
- 1/2 tbsp Dijon mustard
- 1 small clove garlic, finely minced

- 1/2 tsp Worcestershire sauce

- 1/4 lemon (juice of) or 1/2 small lime

- Salt

- Pepper

PREPARATION TIPS

Prep Time	Cook Time	Total Time
10 minutes	8 minutes	18 minutes

Notes:

Adjust the amount of lemon juice based on the desired tanginess. If more juice is added, consider increasing the mayo to maintain the dressing's consistency.

Garlic can be finely chopped or grated using a micro plane zester into the dressing.

Instructions:

1. Assemble all the ingredient

2. Heat a cast-iron pan (or a regular pan) with olive oil over high heat. If the chicken breast is thick, slice it in half

through the middle or pound it to achieve a thinner consistency.

3. Add salt and pepper to the chicken for Seasoning.

4. Place it in the hot pan and reduce the heat to medium-high.

5. Cook each side for 3-4 minutes until golden. Once cooked, place the chicken on a plate or cutting board to rest until ready to serve.

6. While the chicken rests, tear the kale leaves off the thick part of their stems. Bunch the pieces together and chop them into fine shreds or ribbons. Rinse under water and allow the leaves to dry somewhat.

7. Prepare the dressing by whisking all the ingredients together and adding a pinch of salt and pepper.

8. Plate the kale and pour the dressing over the greens. Toss to combine.

9. Cut the chicken on a diagonal and place it on top of the salad. Garnish with shaved parmesan.

10. Serve and enjoy your delicious and healthy Kale Caesar Salad with Grilled Chicken.

Roasted Beet and Goat Cheese Arugula Salad

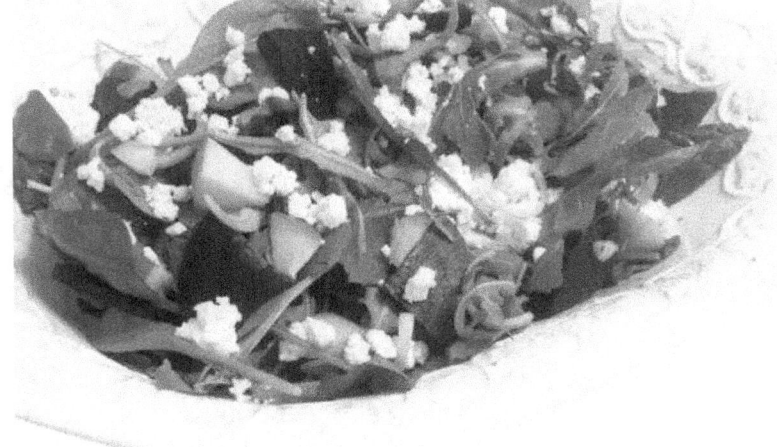

Ingredients:

- 2 beets, thoroughly scrubbed
- 1 bunch of mâche (lamb's lettuce), properly rinsed and dried
- 1 bunch of arugula, well-rinsed and dried
- 2 fresh peaches, peeled, pitted, and sliced
- A single packet (4 ounces) of goat cheese crumbles 1/4 cup of chopped pistachio nuts
- 2 shallots, finely chopped
- 1/4 cup of walnut oil

- 2 tablespoons of balsamic vinegar
- Salt and ground black pepper, to taste

PREPARATION TIPS

Prep Time: 35 mins	Cook Time: 1 hr 20 mins	Additional Time:1hr 10 mins	Total Time: 3 hrs 5 mins

Instruction:

1. Assemble all the ingredient
2. Heat the oven to 375 degrees Fahrenheit, (i.e. 190 degrees Celsius). Wrap each beet in two layers of aluminum foil and arrange them on a baking sheet
3. Bake in the preheated oven until the beets reach a tender consistency, approximately 1 hour and 20 minutes. Allow the beets to cool slightly, and then proceed to remove the skins. Let the beets cool to room temperature or refrigerate until cold, approximately 1 hour.
4. Combine mâche, arugula, thinly sliced cooled beets, peaches, crumbled goat cheese, chopped pistachios, and shallots in a large mixing bowl.
5. Whisk together walnut oil, balsamic vinegar, salt, and pepper in a small bowl until emulsified.
6. Pour the dressing over the salad, toss thoroughly, and serve.

Citrus and Fennel Quinoa Salad

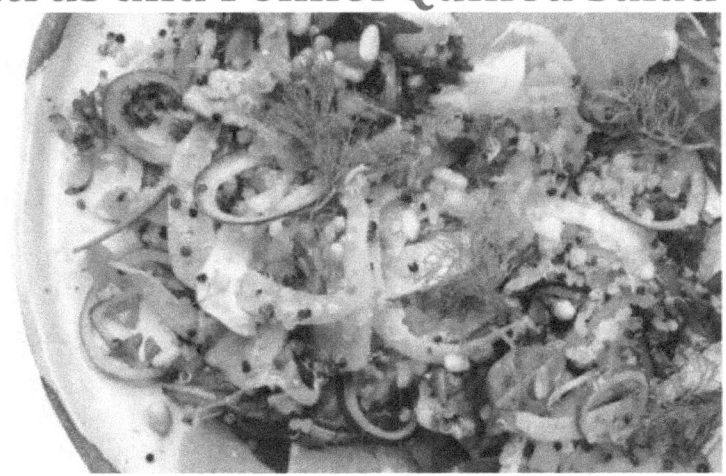

Ingredients:

- 1/2 cup uncooked quinoa
- 2 organic oranges, sliced and peeled
- 1 fennel, trimmed and thinly sliced
- 1 small red onion, thinly sliced
- 3 handfuls of baby arugula leaves
- Handful of parsley, roughly chopped
- 1/3 cup sun-dried apricots, thinly sliced
- 1/4 cup toasted pine nuts
- Juice and zest from one large organic orange
- 1 tablespoon cold-pressed extra-virgin olive oil

- 1 tablespoon pure maple syrup
- 1 tablespoon apple cider vinegar
- Pinch of sea salt

PREPARATION TIPS

Prep time	Cook time	Total Time:	Servings
10 mins	25 mins	35min	4

Procedure:

1. Assemble all the needed ingredient
2. Rinse the quinoa thoroughly to remove its bitter coating, and then place it in a small saucepan.
3. Cover it with water and bring to a boil. Simmer for 14 minutes or until the quinoa is light and fluffy. Set it aside to cool.
4. In a large bowl, combine all the salad ingredients.
5. In a jar, combine the dressing ingredients and shake well to combine. Sprinkle the salad with the dressing and gently toss
6. Arrange the salad on a serving plate and top it with extra pine nuts and parsley.

CHAPTER 5

Hearty Soups and Stews

Hearty soups and stews can contribute to prostate health by incorporating nutrient-rich ingredients known for their potential benefits. Ingredients such as tomatoes, containing lycopene, and cruciferous vegetables like broccoli and cauliflower, rich in sulforaphane, have been associated with a lower risk of prostate issues. Additionally, including lean proteins such as poultry or legumes provides essential amino acids important for overall health. The liquid nature of soups ensures proper hydration, which is vital for maintaining prostate function. Moreover, including whole grains and various vegetables offers dietary fiber, supporting digestive health and potentially influencing prostate well-being. A well-balanced, hearty soup or stew can be a valuable component of a prostate-friendly diet, providing key nutrients and promoting overall wellness.

Lentil and Vegetable Soup

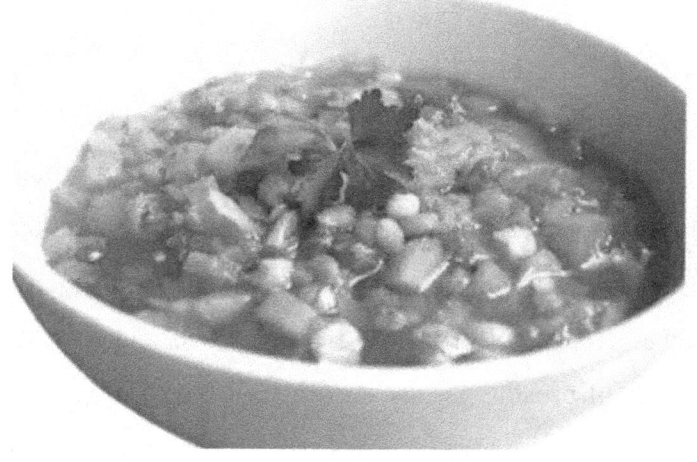

Ingredients:

1/2 cup of red or green lentils

1 cup of chopped onion

1 stalk of celery, chopped

2 cups of shredded cabbage

1 (28 ounces) can of whole peeled tomatoes, chopped

2 cups of chicken broth

3 carrots, chopped

1 clove of garlic, crushed

1 teaspoon salt

1/2 teaspoon ground black pepper

1/4 teaspoon white sugar

1/2 teaspoon dried basil

1/2 teaspoon dried thyme

1/4 teaspoon curry powder

PREPARATION TIPS

Prep Time: 20 mins	Cook Time: 1 hr 30 mins	Additional Time: 1 hr 10 mins
Total Time: 3 hrs	Servings: 6	Yield: 6 to 1 - cup servings

Instructions:

1. Assemble all the ingredient
2. Place the lentils in a stockpot or Dutch oven, adding water to twice the depth of the lentils. Bring to a boil, then reduce the heat and simmer for approximately 15 minutes.
3. Drain and rinse the lentils before returning them to the pot.
4. Add onion, celery, cabbage, tomatoes, chicken broth, carrots, and garlic to the pot.
5. Season with salt, pepper, sugar, basil, thyme, and curry. Simmer for 1 1/2 to 2 hours or until the desired tenderness is achieved.

Note:

For an alternative method, combine all ingredients in a slow cooker. Cook on Low for 8 to 10 hours or on High for about 4 hours, ensuring lentils break down and vegetables reach the desired tenderness.

Minestrone Soup with Whole Grain Pasta

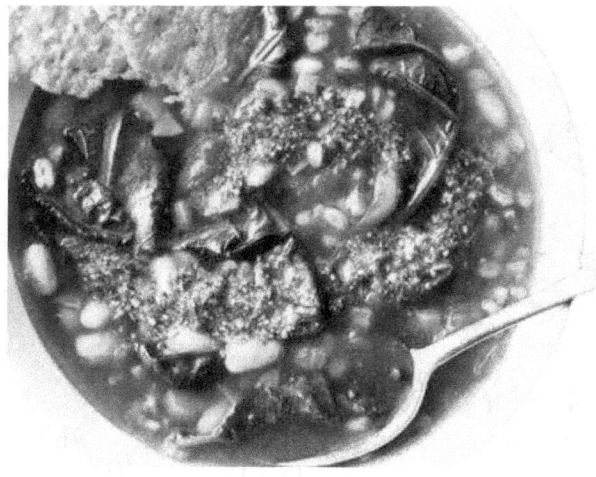

Ingredients:

- 2 tablespoons olive oil
- 1 small yellow onion, finely chopped
- 2 medium carrots, finely chopped
- 2 stalks celery, finely chopped
- 3 cloves garlic, finely chopped

- 1 tablespoon tomato paste
- 1-quart vegetable broth
- 1 can (28 oz.) white beans, drained and rinsed
- 1 can (28 oz.) whole tomatoes, undrained, coarsely crushed
- 1 cup farro
- 1 fresh rosemary sprig
- ¾ teaspoon kosher salt
- ½ teaspoon freshly ground black pepper
- ¾ cup grated Parmesan cheese
- 2 ounces baby kale (about 2 cups)
- Store-bought pesto (optional)

PREPARATION TIPS

Prep Time: 30 mins	Cooking time: 25 mins	Total Time: 55 mins	Yield: 6 serves

Instructions:

1. Assemble all the ingredient
2. Heat 2 tablespoons of olive oil in a large pot or Dutch oven over medium-high heat.

3. Add finely chopped onion, carrots, celery, garlic, and tomato paste. Cook, stirring occasionally, until tomato paste darkens and vegetables are just tender (about 10 minutes).

4. Stir in vegetable broth, drained white beans, undrained crushed tomatoes, and farro, and add the fresh rosemary. Bring the mixture to a boil.

5. Reduce heat to medium and simmer, stirring occasionally, until the farro is tender (about 30 minutes). If the soup is too thick, you can stir in up to 3 cups of water—season with salt and pepper.

6. Meanwhile, in a nonstick skillet, sprinkle an even layer of grated Parmesan cheese to form a large round.

7. Cook without stirring over medium heat until melted and browned (about 3 minutes).

8. Let it cool in the skillet for 3 minutes, then transfer to a plate and break it into pieces.

9. Stir baby kale into the soup and cook until just wilted (about 5 minutes).

10. Garnish each serving with Parmesan crisps and drizzle with pesto if desired.

Turkey and Vegetable Chili

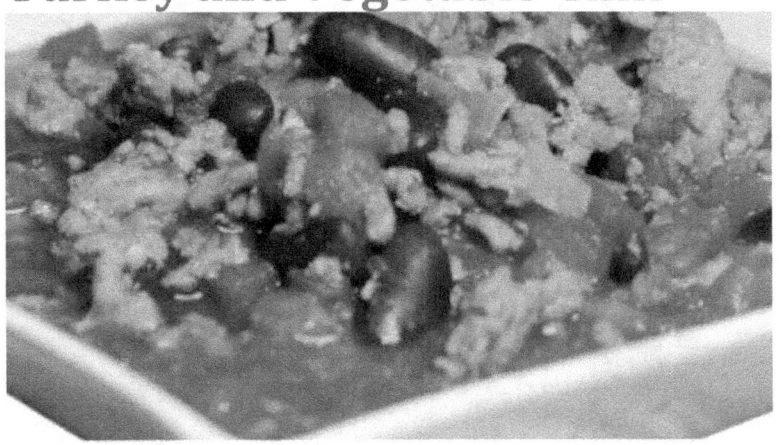

Ingredient List:

- 1 ½ teaspoons of olive oil
- 1 pound of ground turkey
- 1 chopped onion
- 2 cups of water
- 1 can (28 ounces) of crushed tomatoes
- 1 can (16 ounces) of kidney beans, drained, rinsed, and mashed
- 1 tablespoon of minced garlic
- 2 tablespoons of chili powder
- ½ teaspoon of paprika

- ½ teaspoon of dried oregano
- ½ teaspoon of ground cayenne pepper
- ½ teaspoon of ground cumin
- ½ teaspoon of salt
- ½ teaspoon of ground black pepper

PREPARATION TIPS

Prep Time:	Cook Time:	Total Time:	Servings:
15 mins	45 mins	1 hr	8

Instructions:

1. Assemble all the ingredient
2. Heat oil in a big pot on medium heat.
3. Put in turkey and stir until it's uniformly browned, which should take 6 to 8 minutes.
4. Add onion and cook until it becomes tender.
5. Include water and mix in tomatoes, kidney beans, and garlic. Add the chili powder, paprika, oregano, cayenne pepper, cumin, salt, and pepper.
6. Bring it to a boil. Then, lower the heat, cover, and let it simmer for 30 minutes.
7. serve

Mushroom and Barley Soup

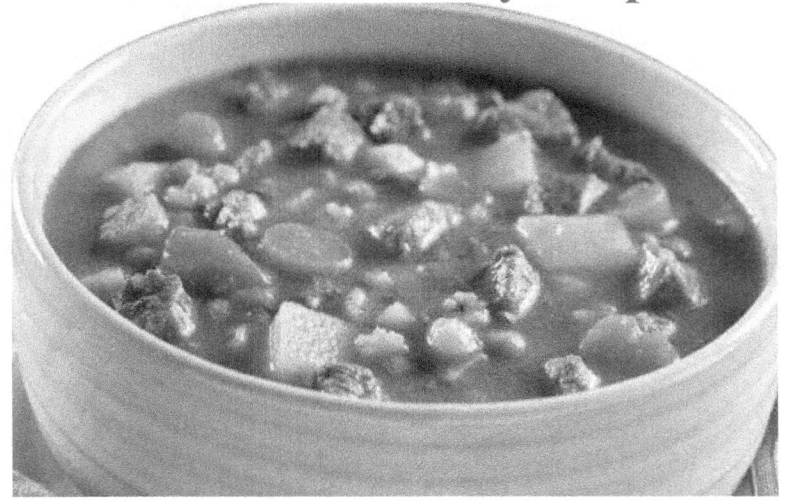

Ingredient List:

- 1/4 cup olive oil
- 1 cup chopped onion
- 3/4 cup diced carrots
- 1/2 cup chopped celery
- 1 teaspoon minced garlic
- 1 pound sliced fresh mushrooms
- 6 cups chicken broth
- 3/4 cup barley
- Salt and pepper to taste

PREPARATION TIPS

Prep Time:	Cook Time:	Total Time:	Servings:
15 mins	55 mins	1 hr 10 mins	6

Instruction:

1. Begin by heating olive oil in a sizable soup pot on medium heat.

2. Introduce onion, carrots, celery, and garlic, stirring until the onion becomes soft and translucent, approximately 5 minutes.

3. Incorporate mushrooms and continue cooking for an additional 3 minutes.

4. Next, pour in chicken broth, add barley, and bring the mixture to a boil. Once boiling, lower the heat to a simmer, cover the pot, and let it cook until the barley reaches a tender consistency, usually lasting around 40 to 50 minutes.

5. Season the soup with salt and pepper and allow it to heat for about 2 minutes.

6. serve

Tomato Basil Soup

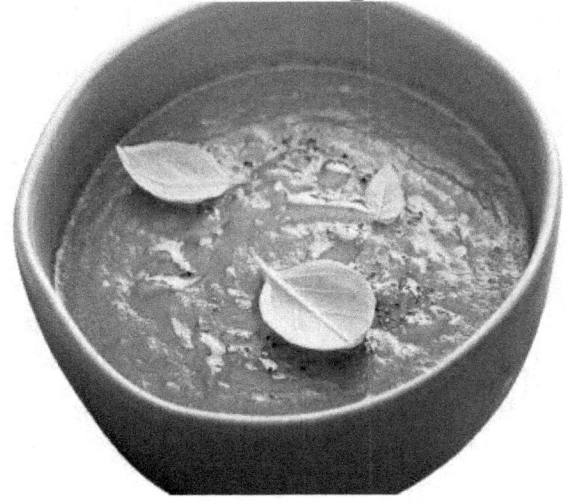

Ingredients:

- 4 pounds of plum tomatoes (Roma tomatoes), cut in half
- 6 cloves of garlic, peeled
- 3 tablespoons of olive oil
- 2 teaspoons of salt, divided
- one teaspoon of freshly ground black pepper
- 1 tablespoon of butter (or dairy-free alternative)
- 2 onions, sliced
- 56 oz whole peeled tomatoes (2 cans of 28 oz each), with juices

- 1 cup of fresh basil leaves, plus more for serving
- 3½ cups of low-sodium vegetable broth (or water, chicken broth, or chicken stock), with more as needed
- 1 teaspoon of granulated sugar (optional)
- 1 teaspoon of red chili flakes, more if desired or less for those sensitive to spicy food
- Heavy cream or coconut milk for serving (optional)
- Croutons or crackers for serving (optional)

PREPARATION TIPS

Prep Time	Cook Time	Total Time	Servings:
10mins	1 hour hr 10 mins	1 hour hr 20 mins	6 servings

Instructions:

1. Roast the tomatoes: Preheat the oven to 425 degrees F. Halve the tomatoes and place them on parchment-lined baking sheets.

2. Add garlic cloves to each sheet. sprinkle with two tablespoons of olive oil and season with salt and pepper. Roast for about 45 minutes (for Roma tomatoes) or 20 minutes (for cherry tomatoes) until the skin is tender.

3. Cook the onions: Heat the remaining tablespoon of olive oil and 1 tablespoon of butter over medium-high heat in a large pot or Dutch oven. Add onions and cook for about 15 minutes until they start to brown and caramelize. Reduce heat if onions begin to burn. Stir frequently.

4. Add the tomatoes: Put canned tomatoes, fresh basil, broth, sugar, and red chili flakes into the pot. Bring to a low boil, and then reduce heat to low and simmer until the roasted tomatoes are ready. Add the oven-roasted tomatoes with their juices and return to a simmer.

5. Simmer: The soup is uncovered over low heat for about 20 minutes.

6. Puree: Carefully blend the homemade tomato soup in batches using a high-speed immersion or handheld food processor. Avoid over-blending.

7. Season and serve: Return the pureed soup to the pot and season with additional salt and pepper to taste. Garnish

with fresh basil, croutons, or a splash of fresh cream if desired. Enjoy!

Notes:

- You can double the number of fresh tomatoes if you don't want to use canned tomatoes.
- To peel tomatoes without roasting, briefly place them in boiling water for 30 seconds until the skin wrinkles. Transfer to ice water to stop cooking and peel the skins.
- Freezing the soup is recommended only if cream or dairy is not added before freezing.
- Adjust the spiciness based on individual preference for red chili flakes.
- Optional garnishes include red pepper flakes, fresh basil, heavy cream, coconut milk, parmesan cheese, homemade croutons, or crackers.

CHAPTER 6

Balanced Smoothies and Snacks

Balanced smoothies and snacks contribute significantly to prostate health by delivering essential nutrients that support overall well-being. Smoothies, crafted with a combination of fruits, vegetables, and protein sources, offer a convenient way to incorporate antioxidants, vitamins, and minerals into the diet. These components play a crucial role in combating oxidative stress, a factor linked to prostate issues. Additionally, snacks such as nuts and yogurt, rich in omega-3 fatty acids, zinc, and probiotics, further enhance the nutritional profile supporting prostate health. Embracing a dietary regimen centered on balanced smoothies and prostate-friendly snacks provides a proactive approach to maintaining optimal prostate function and promoting long-term health.

Green Tea and Berry Smoothie

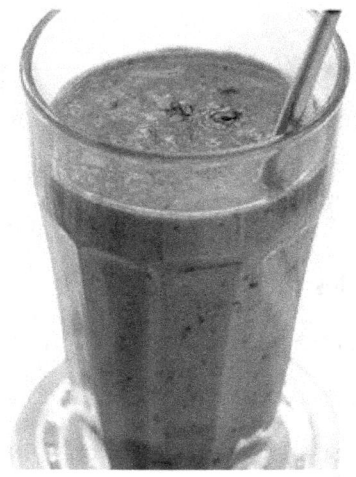

Ingredients:

- 1 cup of green tea, cooled
- 1/2 cup of mixed berries, comprising blueberries, strawberries, and raspberries
- 1/2 banana, frozen
- 1/2 cup of Greek yogurt, plain and low-fat
- 1 tablespoon of ground flaxseeds
- 1 tablespoon of pumpkin seeds
- 1 teaspoon of honey for sweetness (optional)
- Ice cubes (optional for a colder smoothie)

PREPARATION TIPS

Prep time	Cook time	Total Time:	Servings
10 mins	15 mins	25mins	2

Instructions:

1. Brew Green Tea:

Start by brewing a cup of green tea and letting it cool to room temperature.

2. Ingredients:

Gather all the ingredients and ensure they are clean and fresh.

3. Blend Berries and Banana:

In a blender, add the mixed berries and the frozen banana. These berries contain antioxidants that can be beneficial for prostate health.

4. Add Green Tea:

Pour the cooled green tea into the blender. Green tea is rich in polyphenols, associated with potential cancer-fighting properties.

5. Include Greek Yogurt:

Add the Greek yogurt to the blender. Greek yogurt is a good source of protein and probiotics, which can support overall health.

6. Incorporate Flaxseeds:

Sprinkle in the ground flaxseeds. Flaxseeds contain omega-3 fatty acids and fiber, which may contribute to prostate health.

7. Add Pumpkin Seeds:

Toss in the pumpkin seeds. Pumpkin seeds are rich in zinc, an important mineral for prostate function.

Optional Sweetener:

If desired, add a teaspoon of honey for sweetness. Depending on your preference, change the amount.

Blend Until Smooth:

Blend all the ingredients until you achieve a smooth consistency. If you prefer a colder smoothie, you can add a few ice cubes and blend again.

8. Serve and Enjoy:

Pour the smoothie into a glass and enjoy it as a refreshing and prostate-friendly beverage.

Almond Butter and Banana Smoothie

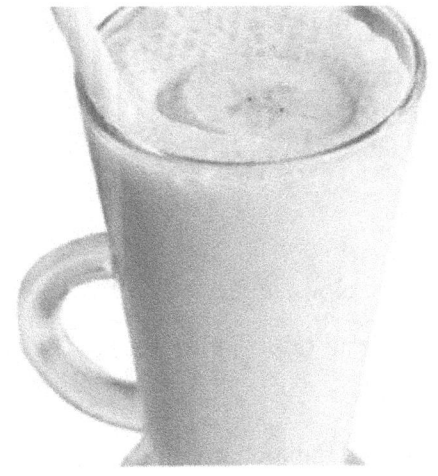

Ingredients:

- 1 medium-sized of ripe banana
- 2 tablespoons of almond butter (unsweetened, no added oils)
- 1 cup of unsweetened almond milk
- 1/2 cup of Greek yogurt (unsweetened)
- one tablespoon of chia seeds (optional)
- Ice cubes (optional)
- Honey or maple syrup for sweetness (optional, based on individual taste)

PREPARATION TIPS

Prep Time:	Cook Time:	Total Time:	Servings:
5 minutes	5 mins	10 minutes	2

Instructions:

1. Peel and slice the ripe banana.
2. Measure the almond butter, almond milk, Greek yogurt, and chia seeds
3. Combine the sliced banana, almond butter, almond milk, Greek yogurt, and chia seeds in a blender.
4. If desired, add a drizzle of honey or maple syrup for sweetness.
5. Blend until smooth. If a thicker consistency is preferred, add ice cubes and blend again.
6. Serve

Notes:

Adjust sweetness based on individual preferences and dietary restrictions.

Greek Yogurt Parfait with Berries and Nuts

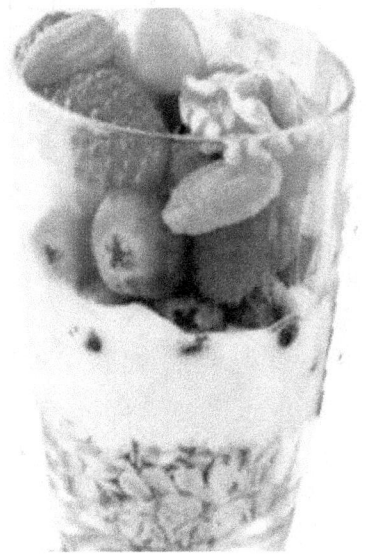

Ingredients:

- Greek Yogurt (unsweetened and low-fat) - 1 cup
- Mixed berries (blueberries, strawberries, raspberries) - 1/2 cup
- Nuts (almonds or walnuts, unsalted) - 1/4 cup
- Honey (optional) - 1 tablespoon for sweetness
- Chia seeds (optional) - 1 tablespoon for added fiber and omega-3 fatty acids

PREPARATION TIPS

Prep time	Cook time	Total Time:	Servings
10 mins	25 mins	35mins	2

Instructions:

1. Select Quality Ingredients:

Choose unsweetened and low-fat Greek yogurt to minimize added sugars and saturated fats. Opt for fresh, organic berries to maximize antioxidant content. Ensure the nuts are unsalted to control sodium intake.

2. Prepare Yogurt Base:

Scoop 1 cup of Greek yogurt into a serving bowl. Greek yogurt is an excellent source of protein, vital for maintaining muscle mass during cancer treatment.

3. Wash and Add Berries:

Wash the mixed berries thoroughly and pat them dry. Add the berries to the yogurt. Berries contain antioxidants that may contribute to overall health and support the immune system.

4. Incorporate Nuts:

Measure 1/4 cup of unsalted nuts (almonds or walnuts) and sprinkle them over the yogurt and berries. Nuts provide healthy fats, such as omega-3 fatty acids, which may be anti-inflammatory.

5. Drizzle with Honey (Optional):

If additional sweetness is desired, drizzle 1 tablespoon of honey over the parfait. However, this step can be omitted for individuals watching their sugar intake.

6. Add Chia Seeds (Optional):

For an extra nutritional boost, sprinkle 1 tablespoon of chia seeds over the parfait. Chia seeds are rich in fiber and omega-3 fatty acids, contributing to digestive health and anti-inflammatory effects.

7. Serve and Enjoy:

Gently mix the ingredients to ensure an even distribution of flavors. Serve the Greek Yogurt Parfait immediately and encourage the patient to enjoy this nutrient-packed and flavorful snack.

Trail Mix with Pumpkin Seeds and Dried Fruit

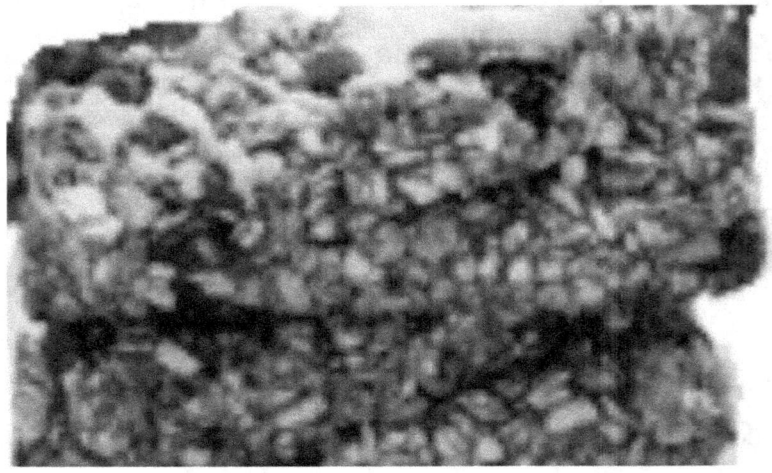

- Ingredients:
- 1 cup of raw pumpkin seeds
- 1 cup of almonds, unsalted
- 1 cup of dried cranberries, unsweetened
- 1 cup of dried apricots, unsulfured and chopped
- 1 cup of walnuts, unsalted
- 1/2 cup of dark chocolate chips, at least 70% cocoa (optional)
- 1/2 teaspoon of sea salt

PREPARATION TIPS

Prep time	Cook time	Total Time:	Servings
20 mins	10 mins	30mins	2

Instructions:

1. Preheat Oven (5 minutes):

Preheat your oven to 325°F (163°C).

2. Toast Pumpkin Seeds (10 minutes):

Spread the raw pumpkin seeds evenly on a baking sheet. Toast them in the preheated oven for about 10 minutes or until they become golden brown and crisp. Be attentive to prevent burning.

3. Prepare Other Ingredients (5 minutes):

While the pumpkin seeds are toasting, chop the dried apricots and gather the remaining ingredients. Ensure the almonds, walnuts, cranberries, and dark chocolate (if using) are ready for mixing.

4. Combine Ingredients (5 minutes):

Combine the toasted pumpkin seeds, almonds, walnuts, dried cranberries, dried apricots, and dark chocolate chips in a large mixing bowl. Add sea salt to taste.

5. Mix Thoroughly:

Gently toss the ingredients until evenly distributed, ensuring a balanced mix of flavors and textures.

6. Store in Airtight Container or serve:

Transfer the trail mix to an airtight container to preserve freshness. Serve or store in a cool, dry place.

Roasted Chickpeas with Mediterranean Spices

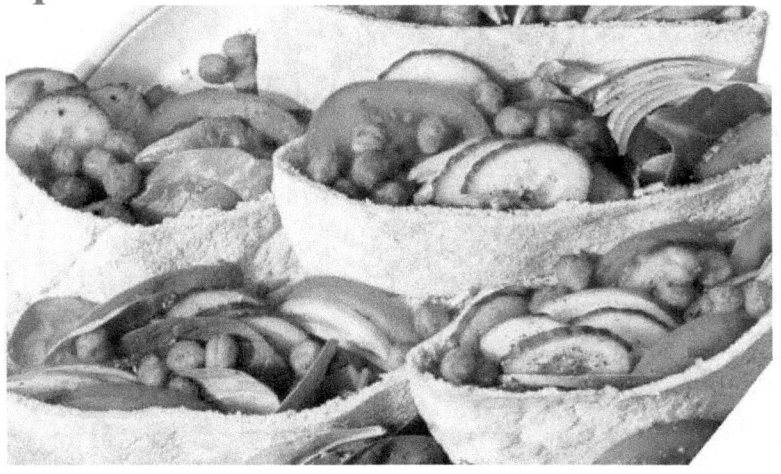

Ingredients:

- One can (15 ounces) of rinsed and drained chickpeas
- 1 tablespoon of olive oil
- 1 tablespoon of paprika
- 1 teaspoon of ground black pepper
- ½ teaspoon of cayenne pepper
- ¼ teaspoon of salt
- 1 cup of tzatziki sauce
- 4 rounds of pita bread (6 inches each)
- 1 medium of tomato, sliced

- ¼ medium of red onion, cut into strips
- 2 leaves of lettuce, chopped

PREPARATION TIPS

Prep Time: 15 mins	Cook Time: 20 mins	Total Time: 35 mins
Servings: 4	Yield: 4	

Instruction:

1. Preheat the oven to 400 degrees F (200 degrees C) and grease a rimmed baking sheet.
2. Pat dry the chickpeas with a paper towel, ensuring the removal of any loose skins. Gently toss the chickpeas with olive oil, paprika, black pepper, cayenne, and salt.
3. Spread the seasoned chickpeas onto the prepared baking sheet.
4. Bake in the preheated oven until the chickpeas are lightly browned but still tender, approximately 20 minutes.

5. While the chickpeas are baking, spread tzatziki sauce inside each pita.

6. Once the chickpeas are done, sprinkle them into the pita pockets and add tomato slices, red onion strips, and chopped lettuce.

7. Serve immediately for a flavorful and satisfying meal.

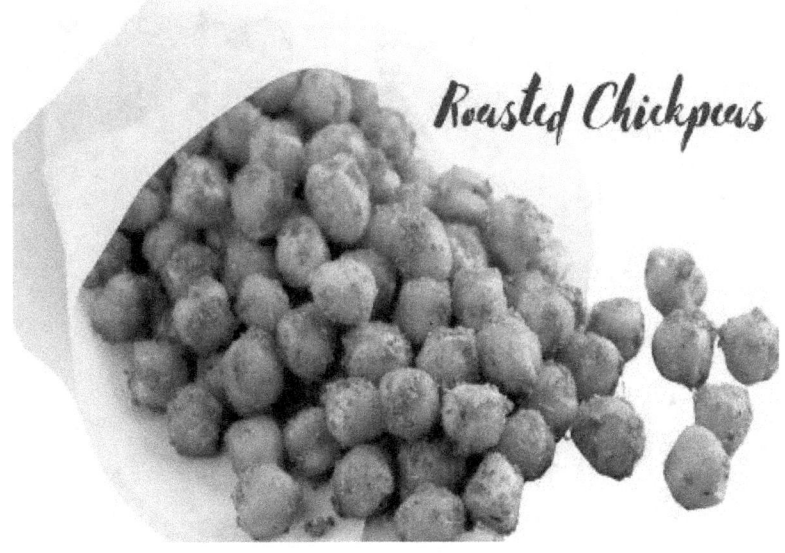

Roasted Chickpeas

Tomato Smoothie

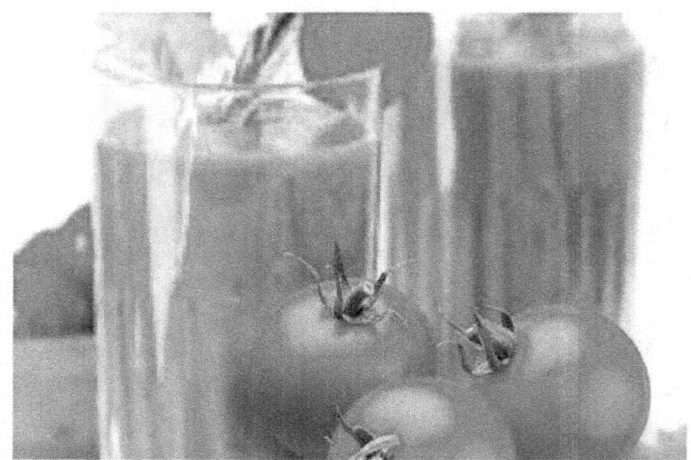

Ingredients

- 3 fresh tomatoes
- 1 cup of tomato juice
- ¼ cup of baby spinach leaves
- 1 big green onion sliced
- 1 celery stalk sliced
- ½ teaspoon of lemon juice
- ¼ teaspoon salt
- ¼ teaspoon of black pepper
- Hot sauce, to taste (optional)
- Ice cube (optionally)

PREPARATION TIPS

Prep Time: 10 mins	Cook Time: 5 mins	Total Time: 15 mins	Serving 2

Instruction

1. Begin by halving the tomatoes and then proceed to dice them into smaller pieces.
2. Place all the specified ingredients into a high-speed blender and proceed to blend until a smooth consistency is achieved.
3. Add the ice cube if desired
4. Taste the mixture and adjust the seasoning according to personal preference.
5. Optionally, incorporate hot sauce to taste, if desired.
6. Serve the prepared mixture promptly in a glass cup.

Notes:

Substitute baby spinach for any green leafy vegetable of your choice such as kale, broccoli etc.

CONCLUSION

In conclusion, "Prostate Cancer Diet Cookbook for Older Men" is a comprehensive guide that offers valuable insights into the dietary considerations essential for managing prostate health in the aging male population. Through meticulous research and evidence-based recommendations, this book underscores the significance of nutrition in preventing and supporting prostate cancer. Providing practical recipes and nutritional guidance tailored specifically for older men equips readers with the tools to make informed choices that can positively impact their well-being.

The culmination of this resource lies in its commitment to empowering individuals with knowledge, encouraging proactive measures, and fostering a holistic approach to health. As readers embrace the principles outlined in this cookbook, they embark on a journey towards improved prostate health, fortified by a well-balanced and purposeful dietary regimen.

This book stands as a testament to the profound impact that informed nutrition can have on mitigating the risks associated with prostate cancer and enhancing the overall quality of life for older men.

To promote health-conscious choices, "Prostate Cancer Diet Cookbook for Older Men" transcends its role as a mere recipe collection, emerging as an indispensable tool for those navigating the complexities of prostate health.

By merging culinary expertise with scientific understanding, this book addresses dietary preferences and strongly emphasizes fostering a proactive and preventive approach to health maintenance.

As readers incorporate the principles conveyed within these pages, they are poised to embark on a transformative journey towards holistic well-being and resilience in the face of prostate-related challenges.

31 DAYS MEAL PLANNER

Meal planner

MONDAY	TUESDAY	WEDNESDAY

THURSDAY	FRIDAY	SHOPPING LIST

SATURDAY	SUNDAY

Notes

Things to avoid

Meal planner

MONDAY	TUESDAY	WEDNESDAY

THURSDAY	FRIDAY	SHOPPING LIST

SATURDAY	SUNDAY

Notes	Things to avoid

Meal planner

MONDAY	TUESDAY	WEDNESDAY

THURSDAY	FRIDAY	SHOPPING LIST
		_____
		_____
		_____
		_____
		_____

SATURDAY	SUNDAY	
		_____
		_____
		_____

Notes	Things to avoid	
		_____
		_____
		_____
		_____

Meal planner

MONDAY	TUESDAY	WEDNESDAY

THURSDAY	FRIDAY	SHOPPING LIST

SATURDAY	SUNDAY	

Notes	Things to avoid	

Meal planner

MONDAY	TUESDAY	WEDNESDAY

THURSDAY	FRIDAY	SHOPPING LIST

SATURDAY	SUNDAY

Notes	Things to avoid

Meal planner

MONDAY	TUESDAY	WEDNESDAY

THURSDAY	FRIDAY	SHOPPING LIST
		_____
		_____
		_____
		_____
		_____

SATURDAY	SUNDAY	_____
		_____
		_____
		_____
		_____
		_____

Notes	Things to avoid	_____
		_____
		_____
		_____

Meal planner

MONDAY	TUESDAY	WEDNESDAY

THURSDAY	FRIDAY	SHOPPING LIST

SATURDAY	SUNDAY	

Notes	Things to avoid	

Meal planner

MONDAY	TUESDAY	WEDNESDAY

THURSDAY	FRIDAY	SHOPPING LIST
		_____
		_____
		_____
		_____
		_____

SATURDAY	SUNDAY	
		_____
		_____
		_____
		_____

Notes	Things to avoid	
		_____
		_____
		_____
		_____

Meal planner

MONDAY	TUESDAY	WEDNESDAY

THURSDAY	FRIDAY	SHOPPING LIST

SATURDAY	SUNDAY

Notes	Things to avoid

Meal planner

MONDAY	TUESDAY	WEDNESDAY

THURSDAY	FRIDAY	SHOPPING LIST
		_____
		_____
		_____
		_____
		_____

SATURDAY	SUNDAY	
		_____
		_____
		_____
		_____

Notes	Things to avoid	
		_____
		_____
		_____
		_____
		_____

Meal planner

MONDAY	TUESDAY	WEDNESDAY

THURSDAY	FRIDAY	SHOPPING LIST

SATURDAY	SUNDAY

Notes	Things to avoid

Meal planner

MONDAY	TUESDAY	WEDNESDAY

THURSDAY	FRIDAY	SHOPPING LIST

SATURDAY	SUNDAY

Notes	Things to avoid

Meal planner

MONDAY	TUESDAY	WEDNESDAY

THURSDAY	FRIDAY	SHOPPING LIST

SATURDAY	SUNDAY	

Notes	Things to avoid	

Meal planner

MONDAY	TUESDAY	WEDNESDAY

THURSDAY	FRIDAY	SHOPPING LIST

SATURDAY	SUNDAY

Notes	Things to avoid

Meal planner

MONDAY	TUESDAY	WEDNESDAY

THURSDAY	FRIDAY	SHOPPING LIST

SATURDAY	SUNDAY

Notes	Things to avoid

Meal planner

MONDAY	TUESDAY	WEDNESDAY

THURSDAY	FRIDAY	SHOPPING LIST

SATURDAY	SUNDAY

Notes	Things to avoid

Meal planner

MONDAY	TUESDAY	WEDNESDAY

THURSDAY	FRIDAY	SHOPPING LIST
		_____
		_____
		_____
		_____
		_____

SATURDAY	SUNDAY	
		_____
		_____
		_____
		_____

Notes	Things to avoid	
		_____
		_____
		_____
		_____
		_____

Meal planner

MONDAY	TUESDAY	WEDNESDAY

THURSDAY	FRIDAY	SHOPPING LIST

SATURDAY	SUNDAY

Notes

Things to avoid

Meal planner

MONDAY	**TUESDAY**	**WEDNESDAY**

THURSDAY	**FRIDAY**	**SHOPPING LIST**

SATURDAY	**SUNDAY**

Notes

Things to avoid

Meal planner

MONDAY	TUESDAY	WEDNESDAY

THURSDAY	FRIDAY	SHOPPING LIST

SATURDAY	SUNDAY

Notes

Things to avoid

Meal planner

MONDAY	TUESDAY	WEDNESDAY

THURSDAY	FRIDAY	SHOPPING LIST

SATURDAY	SUNDAY

Notes	Things to avoid

Meal planner

MONDAY	TUESDAY	WEDNESDAY

THURSDAY	FRIDAY	SHOPPING LIST
		_____
		_____
		_____
		_____
		_____

SATURDAY	SUNDAY	
		_____
		_____
		_____
		_____
		_____

Notes	Things to avoid	
		_____
		_____
		_____
		_____

Meal planner

MONDAY	TUESDAY	WEDNESDAY

THURSDAY	FRIDAY	SHOPPING LIST

SATURDAY	SUNDAY	

Notes	Things to avoid	

Meal planner

MONDAY	TUESDAY	WEDNESDAY

THURSDAY	FRIDAY	SHOPPING LIST

SATURDAY	SUNDAY

Notes	Things to avoid

Meal planner

MONDAY	TUESDAY	WEDNESDAY

THURSDAY	FRIDAY	SHOPPING LIST

SATURDAY	SUNDAY

Notes	Things to avoid

Meal planner

MONDAY	TUESDAY	WEDNESDAY

THURSDAY	FRIDAY	SHOPPING LIST

SATURDAY	SUNDAY

Notes

Things to avoid

Meal planner

MONDAY	TUESDAY	WEDNESDAY

THURSDAY	FRIDAY	SHOPPING LIST

SATURDAY	SUNDAY

Notes	Things to avoid

Meal planner

MONDAY	TUESDAY	WEDNESDAY

THURSDAY	FRIDAY	SHOPPING LIST
		_____
		_____
		_____
		_____
		_____

SATURDAY	SUNDAY	
		_____
		_____
		_____

Notes	Things to avoid	
		_____
		_____
		_____
		_____

Meal planner

MONDAY	TUESDAY	WEDNESDAY

THURSDAY	FRIDAY	SHOPPING LIST

SATURDAY	SUNDAY	

Notes	Things to avoid	

Meal planner

MONDAY	TUESDAY	WEDNESDAY

THURSDAY	FRIDAY	SHOPPING LIST

SATURDAY	SUNDAY

Notes

Things to avoid

Meal planner

MONDAY	TUESDAY	WEDNESDAY

THURSDAY	FRIDAY	SHOPPING LIST

SATURDAY	SUNDAY

Notes	Things to avoid

www.ingramcontent.com/pod-product-compliance
Lightning Source LLC
Chambersburg PA
CBHW071049290526
45795CB00004B/1396